SpringerBriefs in Canc

For further volumes:
http://www.springer.com/series/10786

Paolo Boffetta • Stefania Boccia
Carlo La Vecchia

A Quick Guide to Cancer Epidemiology

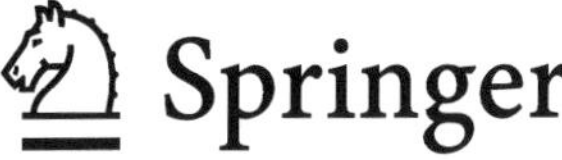

Paolo Boffetta
Mount Sinai School of Medicine
Tisch Cancer Institute
New York, NY, USA

Stefania Boccia
Institute of Public Health Section
of Hygiene
Università Cattolica del Sacro Cuore
Rome, Italy

Carlo La Vecchia
Department of Clinical Sciences
and Community Health
University of Milan
Milan, Italy

ISBN 978-3-319-05067-6 ISBN 978-3-319-05068-3 (eBook)
DOI 10.1007/978-3-319-05068-3
Springer Cham Heidelberg New York Dordrecht London

Library of Congress Control Number: 2014932981

Printed on acid-free paper

Springer is part of Springer Science+Business Media (www.springer.com)

Contents

1 Introduction ... 1

2 Principles of Primary and Secondary Cancer Prevention ... 7
- 2.1 Primary Prevention ... 7
- 2.2 Secondary Prevention ... 8

3 The Global Burden of Neoplasms ... 11

4 Distribution, Causes and Prevention of Individual Neoplasms ... 15
- 4.1 Cancer of the Oral Cavity and Pharynx ... 15
  - 4.1.1 Cancer of the Oral Cavity, Oropharynx and Hypopharynx ... 16
  - 4.1.2 Cancer of the Lip ... 18
  - 4.1.3 Cancer of the Nasopharynx ... 18
  - 4.1.4 Cancer of Salivary Glands ... 19
  - 4.1.5 Prevention of Oral and Pharyngeal Cancers ... 19
- 4.2 Cancer of the Oesophagus ... 19
  - 4.2.1 Adenocarcinoma ... 22
  - 4.2.2 Prevention of Esophageal Cancer ... 22
- 4.3 Cancer of the Stomach ... 23
  - 4.3.1 Prevention of Stomach Cancer ... 24
- 4.4 Cancer of the Intestines ... 25
  - 4.4.1 Cancer of the Small Intestine ... 25
  - 4.4.2 Colon Cancer ... 26
  - 4.4.3 Cancer of the Rectum ... 27
  - 4.4.4 Cancer of the Anus ... 28
  - 4.4.5 Prevention of Intestinal Cancers ... 28
- 4.5 Cancer of the Liver and Biliary Tract ... 29
  - 4.5.1 Hepatocellular Carcinoma ... 29
  - 4.5.2 Other Types of Primary Liver Cancer ... 31

4.5.3 Cancer of Extrahepatic Biliary Ducts 31
4.5.4 Prevention of Liver Cancer and Biliary Tract Cancers 32
4.6 Cancer of the Pancreas 33
4.7 Cancer of the Respiratory Tract 34
4.7.1 Cancer of the Nasal Cavity and the Paranasal Sinuses 34
4.7.2 Cancer of the Larynx 35
4.7.3 Lung Cancer 36
4.7.4 Pleural Mesothelioma 39
4.8 Neoplasms of the Bone and Soft Tissues 41
4.8.1 Bone Cancer 41
4.8.2 Soft Tissue Sarcomas 42
4.9 Cancer of the Skin 42
4.9.1 Non-melanocytic Skin Cancer 43
4.9.2 Prevention of Non-melanocytic Skin Cancer 44
4.9.3 Malignant Melanoma 45
4.9.4 Kaposi's Sarcoma 46
4.10 Cancer of the Breast 46
4.10.1 Prevention of Breast Cancer 50
4.11 Cancer of the Female Genital Organs 51
4.11.1 Cancer of the Uterine Cervix 51
4.11.2 Cancer of the Uterine Corpus 53
4.11.3 Ovarian Cancer 55
4.11.4 Cancer of Vagina and Vulva 56
4.11.5 Choriocarcinoma 57
4.12 Cancer of the Male Genital Organs 57
4.12.1 Prostate Cancer 57
4.12.2 Prevention of Prostate Cancer 59
4.12.3 Testicular Cancer 59
4.12.4 Cancer of the Penis 60
4.13 Cancer of the Urinary Organs 61
4.13.1 Cancer of the Urinary Bladder 61
4.13.2 Cancer of the Kidney 63
4.13.3 Cancer of Renal Pelvis and Ureter 64
4.14 Cancer of the Nervous Organs 65
4.14.1 Cancer of the Eye 65
4.14.2 Cancer of the Nervous System 65
4.15 Cancer of Endocrine Glands 66
4.15.1 Thyroid Cancer 66
4.15.2 Cancer of Other Endocrine Glands 68
4.16 Neoplasms of the Lymphatic and Haematopoietic Organs 68
4.16.1 Hodgkin Lymphoma 69
4.16.2 Non-Hodgkin Lymphoma 70
4.16.3 Multiple Myeloma 71
4.16.4 Leukaemias 72
4.16.5 Prevention of Lymphoid Neoplasms 73
4.17 Childhood and Adolescence Cancers 74

5 Overview of the Major Causes of Human Cancer 77
5.1 Tobacco Smoking 77
5.2 Dietary Factors 78
5.3 Obesity and Physical Exercise 79
5.4 Alcohol Drinking 80
5.5 Infectious Agents 82
5.6 Occupation and Pollution 82
5.7 Reproductive Factors and Exogenous Hormones 84
5.8 Perinatal and Growth Factors 86
5.9 Ionizing and Non-ionizing Radiation 86
5.10 Medical Procedures and Drugs 87
5.11 Genetic Factors 88

6 Conclusions 89

References 91

Abbreviations

EBV Epstein–Barr virus
HBV Hepatitis B virus
HCC Hepatocellular carcinoma
HCV Hepatitis C virus
HIV Human immunodeficiency virus
HL Hodgkin lymphoma
HPV Human papilloma virus
HRT Hormonal replacement therapy
IARC International Agency for Research on Cancer
MOPP Mission oriented protective posture
NHL Non-Hodgkin lymphoma
OC Oral contraceptives
PSA Prostate specific antigen
RB Retinoblastoma
RCT Randomized controlled trials
RR Relative risk
SqCC Squamous cell carcinoma
UBV Ultraviolet radiation
WHO World Health Organisation

Chapter 1
Introduction

Keywords Cancer incidence • Cancer mortality • Cancer trends

Neoplasms include several hundreds of diseases, which can be distinguished by localization, morphology, clinical behaviour and response to therapy.

Benign neoplasms represent localized growths of tissue with predominantly normal characteristics: in most cases they cause minor symptoms and are amenable to surgical therapy. Benign tumours, however, can become clinically important when they occur in organs in which compression is possible and surgery cannot be easily performed (e.g., the brain), and when they produce hormones or other substances with a systemic effect (e.g., epinephrine produced by benign pheochromocytoma). With the exception of benign brain neoplasms, they will not be further addressed.

Malignant neoplasms are characterized by progressive growth of tissue with structural and functional alterations with respect to the normal tissue. In some cases, the alterations can be so important that it becomes difficult to identify the tissue of origin. A peculiarity of most malignant tumours is the ability to migrate and colonize other organs (metastatization) via blood and lymph vessel penetration. The presence and extension of metastases are often the critical factors to determine the success of therapy and the survival of cancer patients.

The pace of growth of malignant neoplasms varies widely, and asymptomatic neoplasms are often found at autopsy of individuals deceased from other causes. The long process of carcinogenesis justifies the efforts to develop and apply screening approaches for early detection of selected subclinical neoplasms in healthy individuals.

Most malignant neoplasms (about 90 %) in adults arise from epithelial tissues and are defined as carcinomas. In practice, however, the terms 'malignant neoplasm', 'malignant tumour' and 'cancer' are used interchangeably. Neoplasms are classified according to the International Classification of Diseases—Oncology (WHO 1990) into topographical categories (according to the organ where the

P. Boffetta et al., *A Quick Guide to Cancer Epidemiology*, SpringerBriefs in Cancer Research, DOI 10.1007/978-3-319-05068-3_1,

neoplasm arises) and morphological categories (according to the characteristics of the cells). More and more often, neoplasms are characterized at the clinical level according to phenotypic aspects (e.g., presence of receptors, expression of genes) and genetic alterations (e.g., mutation in a given gene).

Knowledge about the causes and the possible preventive strategies for malignant neoplasms has greatly advanced during the last decades. This has been largely based on the development of cancer epidemiology. In parallel to the identification of the causes of cancer, primary preventive strategies have been developed. Secondary preventive approaches have also been proposed and in some cases their effectiveness has been evaluated. A careful consideration of the achievements of cancer research, however, suggests that the advancements in knowledge about the causes of cancer have not been followed by an equally important reduction in the burden of cancer. Part of this paradox is explained by the long latency occurring between exposure to carcinogens and development of the clinical disease. Changes in exposure to risk factors are not followed immediately by changes in disease occurrence. The main reason for the gap between knowledge and public health action, however, rests with the cultural, societal and economic aspects of exposure to most carcinogens. The delay in the control of tobacco smoking is the most tragic example of such a gap.

The carcinogenic process may be represented as a succession of stages, taking place in the time span from first exposure to a carcinogenic agent to the appearance of clinical cancer. In its simplest form, as first brought out in mouse skin carcinogenesis experiments, the multistage process reduces to two stages: an irreversible 'initiation' stage inducing malignant cells, and a 'promotion' stage which propagates these cells into a malignant growth. A third stage of 'progression', characterized by an increased rate of growth and metastases, as well as an increase in chromosomal changes in the cell, has also been observed. Formal statistical multistage models of carcinogenesis have provided a useful framework to interpret on a common basis of (postulated) mechanism both experimental and epidemiological observations. As the stages are assumed to occur in a specific sequence, some may be described as 'early' and some as 'late'. Epidemiological observations indicate that, for example, smoking has both an early stage effect, as indicated by the existence of a minimum interval of several years before an increase in risk of lung cancer becomes manifest, and a late stage effect, as indicated by the decrease in risk (with respect to continuous smokers) soon after stopping smoking.

In contrast, asbestos has essentially an early stage effect in the process of pleural (mesothelioma) carcinogenesis, since a latency of several decades is required before an effect is evident, and stopping exposure does not lead to a substantial reduction of risk (La Vecchia and Boffetta 2012).

The identification of the determinants of cancer relies on two complementary approaches, the epidemiological and the experimental. The epidemiological approach has produced both general and specific evidence for the role of different types of agents in cancer causation. The evidence of a more general nature derives from the observations of considerable variation of the incidence rates of most cancers in different populations, defined according to geographical area. Table 1.1

Table 1.1 Ratio of the highest to lowest age-standardized rate in the ranking of country-specific estimated age-standardized incidence rates of selected cancers (Ferlay et al. 2013)

	Men	Women
Cancer	Highest/lowest	Highest/lowest
All cancer, excluding skin	6.80	4.72
Oral cavity	75.75	105.50
Thyroid	173.00	886.00
Nasopharynx	106.00	39.00
Other pharynx	149.00	33.00
Larynx	47.33	30.00
Esophagus	94.00	208.00
Stomach	47.92	49.40
Colorectum	41.07	35.80
Liver	81.50	87.29
Pancreas	39.67	79.00
Gall bladder	78.00	128.00
Lung	191.50	188.00
Melanoma	405.00	331.00
Breast		24.33
Cervix		37.95
Corpus uteri		341.00
Ovary		18.63
Prostate	189.33	
Testis	122.00	
Bladder	103.33	24.67
Kidney	241.00	105.00
Brain, nervous system	127.00	107.00
Kaposi sarcoma	464.00	236.00
Non Hodgkin's lymphoma	36.20	36.50

reports the ratio of the 80th to the 20th percentile of the ranking of country-specific incidence rates of selected cancers, as estimated in the GLOBOCAN 2008 project (Ferlay et al. 2010b). For all gender-specific rates but one, the ratio is above 2, and for several neoplasms it is close to 10. This comparison is based on stable figures, but masks ever larger variations among very-high-risk and very-low-risk areas, which for many neoplasms may reach 100- or even 1,000-fold differences. Variations are also shown within countries or according to other characteristics such as ethnic group, religion, social class. For instance, when contrasted with other religious groups, the Mormons of Utah and the Seventh-Day Adventists of California exhibit low rates for cancers of the respiratory, gastrointestinal and genital systems. This marked variation in rates according to different axes of exploration is unlikely to be explained chiefly by concomitant genetic variations, and points to the role of life-style determinants.

In addition, the observation of changes of incidence in migrant groups after they have moved to a new living environment suggests a major role of non-genetic

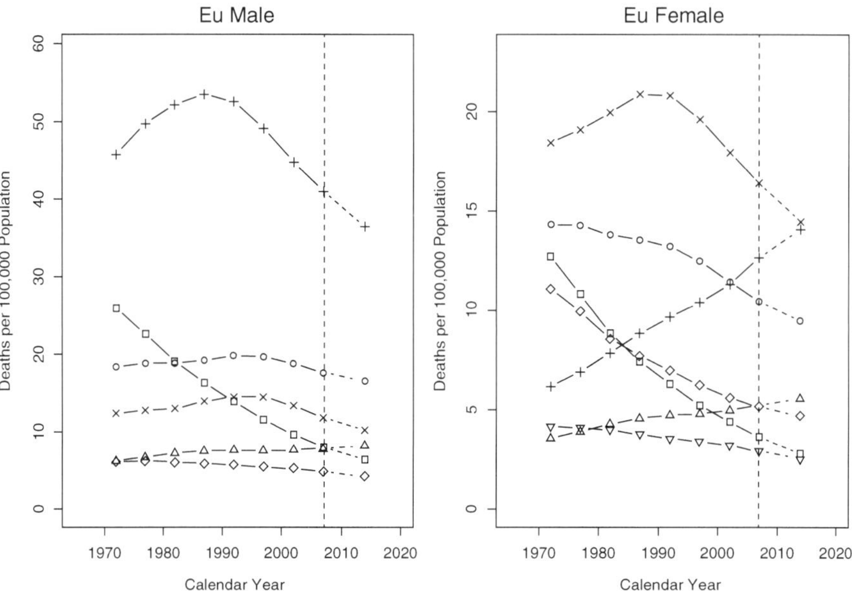

Fig. 1.1 Age-standardized (world population) EU male and female cancer mortalities in quinquennia from 1970–1974 to 2005–2009 and the predicted rates for 2013 (modified) (Malvezzi et al. 2014)

factors. Of course, migrants are selected members of a population and they are likely to be in several aspects different from both their population of origin and from the population of the receiving countries. This demands caution when interpreting data from migrant studies, particularly when dealing with minor differences in rates. However, studies like those of Japanese migrants to Hawaii show an assimilation of their cancer incidence rates to the pattern of Whites, with the emergence of large differences in respect to the rates in Japan, which appears hard to explain solely on the basis of selective factors.

Changes in incidence rates in time, particularly when they take place over a few decades are incompatible with a genetic explanation, as changes in the genes of a population pool require longer intervals. Recorded incidence rates are affected by diagnostic changes and primary prevention programmes (see Sect. 2.1). Mortality rates are, in addition, affected by changes in treatment effectiveness and secondary prevention programmes (see Sect. 2.2); however, marked trends like the one for lung cancer mortality (Fig. 1.1) (Malvezzi et al. 2013a) are most likely to reflect real changes in cancer rates, pointing to the importance of the control of environmental factors.

Analytical studies (case–control and cohort) have shown the causal role of specific exposures in the aetiology of several malignant neoplasms. One limitation of the epidemiological approach, which may prove of critical importance in trying to detect comparatively small increases in risk, as in the case of environmental pollutants, is that even in the best conditions it is impossible to confidently identify by epidemiological means an increase in risk smaller than say 10–20 % (and serious problems arise in the interpretation of increases below 50 %), as the biases inherent in any observational study are of at least this order of magnitude (Adami et al. 2008).

Genetic determinants of cancer have also been demonstrated. As discussed in Sect. 5.11 and in the site specific cancer sections (Chap. 4), several inherited conditions carry a very high risk of one or several cancers. High-penetrance genes are identified through family-based and other linkage studies. These conditions, however, are rare and explain only a small proportion of human cancers. Genetic factors, however, are likely to play an important role in interacting with non-genetic factors to determine individual susceptibility to cancer.

The understanding of the molecular and cellular mechanisms of carcinogenesis has greatly advanced in recent years. According to a widely accepted model, cells have to acquire at least six characteristics to become fully malignant (Hanahan and Weinberg 2011). These include the ability to produce growth signals (several known oncogenes mimic growth signaling), the lack of sensitivity to antigrowth signals (the Retinoblastoma (RB) protein and its homologues play a key role in the ability of the cell to decide whether to proliferate, to be quiescent, or to enter into a post-mitotic state, based on external signaling), resistance towards programmed cell death or apoptosis (in many cases via inactivation of the p53 protein), immortalization (normal cells have a limited replication potential, that is related to the length of the telomeres: in malignant cells overexpression of telomerases circumvents it), stimulation of blood vessel production (by changing the balance of angiogenesis inducers and countervailing inhibitors), and ability to invade and metastasize. The acquisition of these neoplastic characteristics typically occurs by alterations of relevant genes, but an inability to maintain genomic integrity (so-called genomic instability, which includes reduced ability to repair DNA damage) is an additional feature of malignant cells, as accumulation of random mutations in genes involved in all the functions mentioned above would be a too rare event for the development of cancer during the normal lifespan. Inflammation also fosters multiple hallmark functions, and consequently promotes carcinogenesis. A final point to consider is the heterogeneity of neoplastic genetic alterations: the acquisition of the different biological capabilities of the neoplastic cell can appear at different times, and the particular sequence in which capabilities are acquired can vary widely, even among the same type of tumors. In addition, tumours contain a repertoire of normal cells, which contribute to create the tumor microenvironment.

The identification of carcinogens via the laboratory relies on three types of tests: (1) long-term (often lifetime) carcinogenicity tests in experimental animals, most commonly rodents (mice, rats, hamsters), (2) short-term tests assessing the effect of chemical agents on a variety of endpoints belonging to three general classes: DNA damage, mutagenicity and chromosome damage, and (3) mechanistic test, aimed at identifying the intermediate steps in the compound-specific carcinogenic process.

These tests are valuable to the extent that such effects may reflect underlying events in the carcinogenic process. Indeed, consistent positivity in tests measuring DNA damage, mutagenicity and chromosomal damage is usually regarded as indicating potential carcinogenicity of the tested agent. In addition, a number of factors, including hormones and overweight/obesity, show carcinogenic effects through nongenotoxic pathways, for which mechanisms of carcinogenesis are less well defined and their biomarkers are sparse (Boffetta and Islami 2013).

Results of laboratory tests constitute useful supporting evidence when adequate epidemiological data for the carcinogenicity of an environmental agent exist (for example, vinyl chloride), but they become all the more essential when the epidemiological evidence is non-existent or inadequate in quality or in quantity. In the latter case, although no universally accepted criteria exist to automatically translate data from long-term animal tests or short-term tests in terms of cancer risk in humans, an evaluation of the risk can be made on a judgmental basis using all available scientific evidence. This policy has been applied by the International Agency for Research on Cancer (IARC) in a systematic programme of evaluation of the carcinogenic risk of chemicals to man. Within this programme of IARC Monographs, agents are classified in group 1 (established human carcinogen), 2A (probable human carcinogens), 2B (possible human carcinogens) and 3 (not classifiable as to carcinogenicity to humans) (http://monographs.iarc.fr/index.php). Agents are commonly classified in group 1 when the evidence of their carcinogenicity in humans, derived from epidemiological studies, is considered sufficient, and are classified in group 2A when the evidence in humans is limited and the agent is an experimental carcinogen. Agents in group 2B include mainly experimental carcinogens for which the human evidence is inadequate or non-existent. Between 1972 and 2013, 109 volumes presenting evaluations (and re-evaluations) for 970 chemical, physical and biological agents and groups of agents, as well as exposure circumstances such as occupations, have been published. A total of 113 agents have been classified in group 1, 66 in group 2A, and 285 in group 2B, 500 in group 3 and only 1 in group 4. The complete list of agents, with their evaluations can be found on the Monographs web site.

Chapter 2
Principles of Primary and Secondary Cancer Prevention

Keywords Primary prevention • Secondary prevention

2.1 Primary Prevention

The main goal of primary prevention of cancer is to reduce the incidence through the reduction of exposure to risk factors for cancer at population level. Where feasible, primary prevention programmes are demonstrated to be largely cost-effective, i.e. the reduction of the burden of disease is achieved with a reasonable money investment, while this is not always the case for secondary prevention programmes.

Many determinants of malignant neoplasms, including UV radiation, ionizing radiation, tobacco smoking, alcohol drinking, a number of viruses and parasites, and a number of chemicals, industrial processes and occupational exposures, are sufficiently well established to constitute logical priorities for preventive action. Two more reasons add weight to this priority: some of the agents are responsible for sizeable proportions of the cancers occurring today, and for many agents it is in principle feasible to reduce or even to completely eliminate exposure. If this is taken as the objective of preventive action, some practical points are helpful in guiding such action.

First, although epidemiological data in most cases do not allow a direct estimate of the risk of cancer at low doses, it is reasonable (at least from a preventive point of view) to assume that the dose (exposure)-risk relationships for agents acting through damage to DNA is linear with no threshold (Peto et al. 1991). Second, the carcinogenic effect is not equally dependent on the dose rate (dose per unit of time) and on duration of exposure. For example, in regular smokers, the incidence rate of lung cancer depends more strongly on duration of exposure, increasing with the fourth power of it, than on dose rate, increasing only with the first or second power of it (Peto 1977).

P. Boffetta et al., *A Quick Guide to Cancer Epidemiology*, SpringerBriefs in Cancer Research, DOI 10.1007/978-3-319-05068-3_2, © The Author(s) 2014

The attribution of causality to specific agents (as done when, for instance, smoking is said to be the cause of some 30 % of all cancers deaths; see Sect. 5.1) is complicated by their interactive effects. This is particularly relevant when considering the relative effectiveness of removing (or reducing) exposure to one of two (or more) jointly-acting agents. Whenever a positive interaction (synergism) occurs between two (or more) hazardous exposures, there is an enlarged possibility of preventive action; the effect of the joint exposure can be attacked in two (or more) ways, each requiring the removal or reduction of one of the exposures; moreover, the larger the size of the interaction relative to the total effect, the more these ways of attack tend to become equal in effectiveness.

Finally, reducing exposure to carcinogens can be implemented in two major ways: by elimination of the carcinogen or its substitution with a non-carcinogen, or by impeding by various means the contact between the carcinogen and people. Reduction of exposure depends in each case on technical and economical considerations.

Cancer prevention strategies have evolved from a predominant environmental and lifestyle approach to a model that matches individual-oriented actions with public health interventions. Advances in identifying, developing, and testing agents with the potential either to prevent cancer initiation, or to inhibit or reverse the progression of initiated lesions support this approach. Encouraging laboratory and epidemiologic studies, along with studies of secondary endpoints in prevention trials, have provided a scientific rationale for the hypothesis promising results have been reported for various types of cancer, in particular among high-risk individuals (Greenwald 2005; Boffetta and La Vecchia 2009; Zhang et al. 2014).

2.2 Secondary Prevention

Given the limitations still constraining the primary prevention of many cancers, early detection needs to be considered as a secondary and alternative option, based on the reasonable expectation that the earlier the diagnosis and the stage at which a malignancy is discovered, the better the prognosis. This implies that an effective treatment for the disease exists and that the less advanced the cancer at the pre-clinical stage, the better the scope for treatment, and the better the prognosis. This latter aspect cannot be taken for granted.

Before a screening programme can be adopted on a large scale, a number of other requirements need to be fulfilled. First of all, a screening test (that is, a relatively simple and rapid test aimed at the presumptive identification of pre-clinical disease) must be available that is capable of correctly identifying cases and non-cases. In other words, both sensitivity and specificity should be high, approaching 100 %. While high sensitivity is obviously important, given that the very purpose of screening is to pick up, if possible, all cases of a cancer in its detectable pre-clinical phase, it is specificity that plays a dominant role in the practical utilization of the test within a defined population. As the prevalence of a pre-clinical cancer to be screened in well-defined populations is often in the range of 1–10 per 1,000, if a test is used with a specificity of 95 %, then 5 % of results will be false-positives. In other words, for every case which will turn out at the diagnostic work-up to be a true cancer (assuming 100 % sensitivity), there will be 5–50 cases falsely identified as such and ultimately found not to be cancers. This situation is likely to prove unacceptable due to too high psychological and economical costs. One solution is an increase in specificity, for example by developing better tests or combinations of tests, or by changing the criterion of positivity of a given test to make it more stringent (this necessarily decreases sensitivity). In addition, one might select populations with relatively high prevalence of the cancer ('high-risk' groups), so as to increase the number of the true positives. Whatever the group on which the programme operates, additional requirements are that the test is safe, easily and rapidly applicable, and acceptable in a broad sense to the population to be examined. It has also to be cheap, but what is or is not cheap is better evaluated within a cost-effectiveness analysis of different ways of preventing a cancer case or death, an issue not further discussed here.

If these requirements are met, still little is known about the possible net benefit in outcome deriving from the screening programme (in fact, screening test plus diagnostic work-up plus treatment, as applied in a given population). To evaluate benefit, several measures of outcome can be assessed. An early one, useful but not sufficient, is the distribution by stage of the detected cancer cases which, if the programme is ultimately to be beneficial, should be shifted to earlier, less invasive stages of the disease in comparison with the distribution of the cases discovered through ordinary medical care. A second measure of outcome is the survival of cases detected at screening compared with the survival of cases detected through ordinary medical care. This is a superficially attractive but usually equivocal criterion, to the extent that a screening may only advance the time of diagnosis (and therefore the apparent survival time), without postponing the time of death ('lead-time bias'). A final outcome (and the main test of the programme) is the site-specific cancer mortality in the screened population compared with the mortality in the unscreened population.

Correct, unbiased comparison of this outcome, and thus unbiased measure of the effect of the screening programme, should in principle be made within the framework of a randomized controlled trial, in which two groups of subjects are randomly allocated to the screening programme and to no screening (that is, receiving only the existing medical care system) or to two alternative screening programmes, for instance, entailing different tests or different intervals between periodical examinations. However, largely due to pressures to adopt on a large scale screening programmes hoped to be effective, a situation has often arisen where withholding screening to a group has been regarded as unethical or socially unacceptable, thus preventing the conduct of a proper experiment. Very few randomized trials evaluating the effectiveness of screening programmes are available. Comparisons made through non-randomized experiments or through observational studies.

In addition to lead-time bias, three types of bias are peculiar to the assessment of screening programmes. Because of self-selection, persons who elect to receive early detection may be different from those who do not: for instance, they may belong to better educated classes, be generally healthier and health conscious, and this could produce a longer survival independent of any effect of early detection. In addition, cancers with longer pre-clinical phases, which may mean less biological aggressiveness and better prognosis, are, in any case, more likely to be intercepted by a programme of periodical screening than cancers with a short pre-clinical phase, and a rapid, aggressive clinical course (length bias). Finally, because of criteria of positivity adopted to maximize yield of early cases, a number of lesions which in fact would never become malignant growths are included as 'cases', thus falsely improve the survival statistics (over-diagnosis bias).

Chemoprevention can also be considered for primary and secondary prevention of cancer, but data are negative or inconsistent for most micronutrients or other substances considered. Data are however more promising for aspirin, see Sect. 5.10.

Chapter 3
The Global Burden of Neoplasms

Keywords Cancer incidence • Cancer causes

The number of new cases of cancer which occurred worldwide in 2008 has been estimated at about 12,700,000 (Table 3.1) (Ferlay et al. 2010a). Of these, 6,600,000 occurred in men and 6,000,000 in women. About 5,600,000 cases occurred in high-resource countries (North America, Japan, Europe including Russia, Australia and New Zealand) and 7,100,000 in low- and medium-resource countries. Among men, lung, stomach, colorectal, prostate and liver cancers are the most common malignant neoplasms (Fig. 3.1), while breast, colorectal, cervical, lung and stomach are the most common neoplasms among women (Fig. 3.2).

The number of deaths from cancer was estimated at about 7,600,000 in 2008 (Table 3.2) (Ferlay et al. 2010a). No global estimates of survival from cancer are available: data from selected cancer registries suggest wide disparities between high- and low-resource countries for neoplasms with effective but expensive treatment, such as leukaemia, while the gap is narrow for neoplasms without an effective therapy, such as lung cancer (Baili et al. 2008; Sant et al. 2009; Sankaranarayanan et al. 2011) (Fig. 3.3). The overall 5-year survival of cases diagnosed during 1995–1999 in 23 European countries was 49.6 % (Sant et al. 2009).

One complementary approach in assessing the global burden of neoplasms is to estimate the loss in disability-adjusted life-years. This indicator weighs the years of life with disability and add them to the years lost because of premature death. An estimate for 2008 resulted in about 169,000,000 disability-adjusted life-years (DALYs) lost worldwide because of malignant neoplasms. In absolute terms, Asia and Europe contributed to 73 % of DALYs lost because of cancer, and China for 25 %. Lung, liver, breast, stomach, colorectal, cervical, and oesophageal cancers, and leukemia had the highest proportion of DALYs with a combined contribution of 65 % to the total cancer burden (Soerjomataram et al. 2012).

P. Boffetta et al., *A Quick Guide to Cancer Epidemiology*, SpringerBriefs in Cancer Research, DOI 10.1007/978-3-319-05068-3_3,

Table 3.1 Estimated number of new cases of cancer (incidence) and of cancer deaths (mortality) in 2002, by gender and geographical area (Ferlay et al. 2013)[a]

	Men	Women	Total
Incidence			
High-income countries	3,245,000	2,830,000	6,075,000
Low- and middle-income countries	4,185,000	3,830,000	8,015,000
Total	7,430,000	6,660,000	14,090,000
Mortality			
High-income countries	1,590,000	1,290,000	2,880,000
Low- and middle-income countries	3,060,000	2,260,000	5,320,000
Total	4,650,000	3,550,000	8,200,000

[a]The sum of strata does not necessarily round up to the total due to rounding approximation

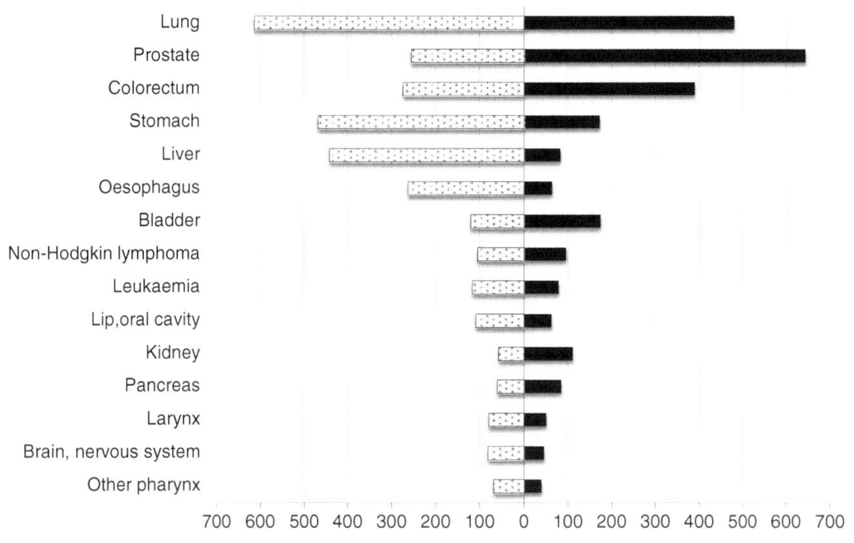

Fig. 3.1 Estimated number of new cancer cases (×1,000), 2002—men (Ferlay et al. 2010b)

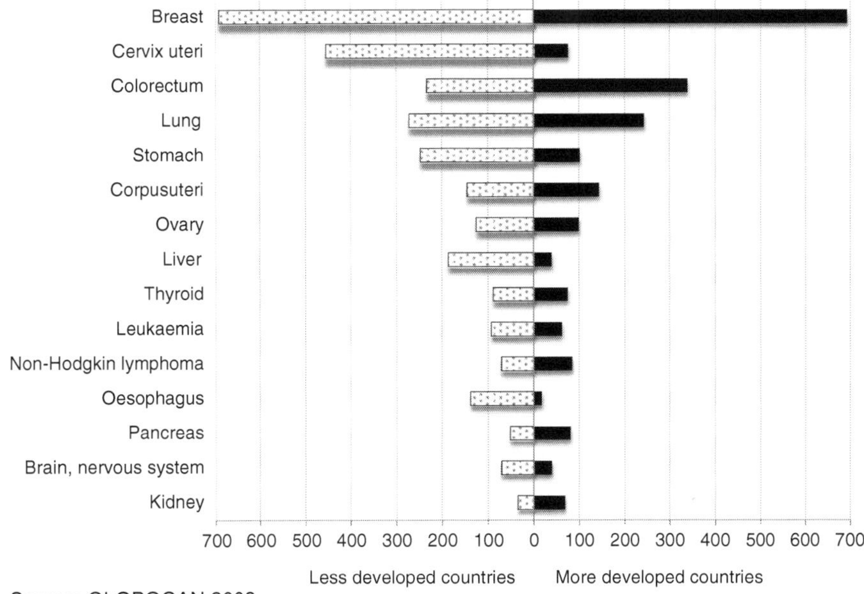

Fig. 3.2 Estimated number of new cancer cases (×1,000), 2002—women (Ferlay et al. 2010b)

Table 3.2 Estimate of the proportion of cancers attributable to major risk factors in the United Kingdom (Doll and Peto 2005)

	Attributable proportion (%)		
Risk factor	Best estimate	Range of acceptable estimates	Avoidable in practice (%)
Tobacco smoking	30	27–33	30
Alcohol drinking	6	4–8	6[a]
Ionizing radiation	5	4–6	<1
Ultraviolet light	1	1	<1
Infections	5	4–15	1
Medical drugs	<1	0–1	<1
Occupation	2	1–5	<1
Pollution	2	1–5	<1
Diet and obesity	25	15–35	2
Reproduction and other hormonal factors	15	10–20	<1
Physical inactivity	<1	0–1	<1

[a]Total avoidance of alcohol would increase overall mortality as the increase in cardiovascular mortality would exceed the reduction in cancer mortality

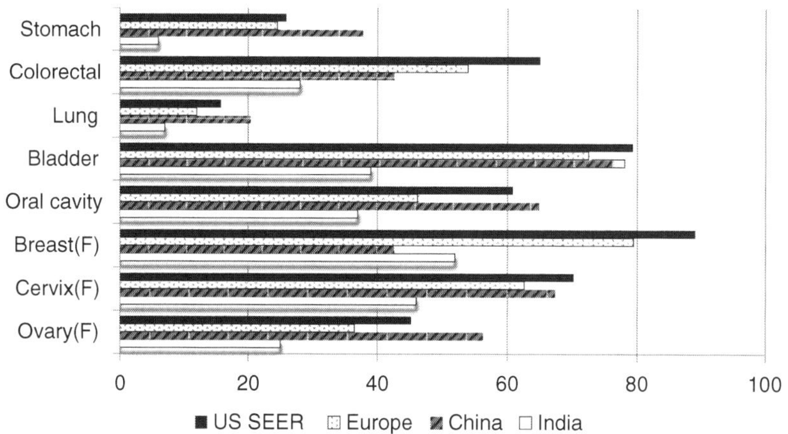

Source: American Cancer Society. *Global Cancer Facts & Figures 2nd Edition.*
Sant M, Allemani C, Santaquilani M, Knijn A, Marchesi F, Capocaccia R; EUROCARE Working Group. EUROCARE-4. Survival of cancer patients diagnosed in 1995-1999. Results and commentary. Eur J Cancer. 2009 Apr;45(6):931-91.

Fig. 3.3 Five-year relative survival from cancer in selected populations (Baili et al. 2008; Sant et al. 2009; Sankaranarayanan et al. 2011)

Chapter 4
Distribution, Causes and Prevention of Individual Neoplasms

Keywords Biliary tract • Bone • Breast • Endocrine glands • Female genital organs • Haematopoietic organs • Intestine • Liver • Lymphatic organs • Male genital organs • Neoplasms • Nervous organs • Oesophagus • Oral cavity • Pancreas • Pharynx • Respiratory tract • Skin • Soft tissues • Stomach • Urinary organs

This section includes a systematic review of the descriptive epidemiology of the most important malignant neoplasms. It also includes an overview of the current state of knowledge about the risk factors and the strategies for primary and secondary prevention. We chose a global approach, which excludes important local aspects of the descriptive epidemiology, the aetiology and the prevention of neoplasms. All incidence and mortality rates are standardized to the world population. We report estimates for 2008 (Ferlay et al. 2010a, b) since more recent data are available only for selected regions and countries.

4.1 Cancer of the Oral Cavity and Pharynx

Tumours of the oral cavity and the pharynx comprise a broad group of different malignant neoplasms. Cancers of the oral cavity, oropharynx (including the tonsil) and hypopharynx are usually considered as a group, because of shared descriptive characteristics and risk factors, while neoplasms arising from the lip, nasopharynx and salivary glands are treated separately, because of differences in aetiological factors.

An estimated 400,000 new cases of cancers of the oral cavity and pharynx occurred in the world in 2008, two-thirds of which in low- and middle-income countries. The estimated number of deaths is 220,000 (170,000 in low- and middle-income countries) (Ferlay et al. 2010a).

P. Boffetta et al., *A Quick Guide to Cancer Epidemiology*, SpringerBriefs in Cancer Research, DOI 10.1007/978-3-319-05068-3_4,

4.1.1 Cancer of the Oral Cavity, Oropharynx and Hypopharynx

The incidence of cancers of the oral cavity and pharynx varies over tenfold between high-risk areas (>20/100,000 in men; Central and Southern Europe and India) and low-risk areas (<2/100,000 in men; China and Arabic countries) (Forman et al. 2013). In all populations, rates in men exceed those in women by a factor of 2–5. Incidence rates have increased in Europe and the Americas until the late 1980s had have levelled off or declined in most countries over the last decade. When looking at subsites within the oral cavity and the pharynx, cancer of the oropharynx and hypopharynx account for as many or more cases than cancer of the oral cavity in high-risk European populations, while cancers of the tongue, floor of the mouth and other parts of the oral cavity represent the majority of cases in India and the USA.

Tobacco and alcohol are the more important risk factor for cancer of the oral cavity and pharynx. In Western populations, smoking represents the main use of tobacco, and Relative Risk (RR) of oral cancer among smokers, as compared to non-smokers, are in the order of 3–10. The risk is higher for heavy smokers, long-term smokers, smokers of black tobacco or high-tar cigarettes. Cigar and pipe smoking also poses a risk, while stopping smoking is followed by a decrease in risk. In India, chewing of products containing tobacco is the main risk factor for oral cancer, although bidi and cigarette smoking also contribute to the risk. The evidence of a role of smokeless tobacco products in other countries remains controversial (Boffetta et al. 2008).

Consumption of alcoholic beverages increases the risk of oral and pharyngeal cancer. Relative to abstainers and very light drinkers, the RR in heavy drinkers is in the order of 10. The effects of tobacco smoking and alcohol drinking are multiplicative or over multiplicative, that is, the effect of exposure to both is close to or greater than the product of their individual effects (Fig. 4.1). The combined effect of tobacco smoking and alcohol drinking accounts for almost 80 % of cancers of the oral cavity and pharynx in most high-risk populations. Similarly, alcohol drinking and tobacco chewing and smoking and their combination are responsible for a large proportion of these cancers in India.

With reference to alcohol drinking, additional issues are worth discussing. First, oral cancer risks show a clear decline after stopping smoking, but the pattern of risk after stopping drinking remains unclear, though it appears that an appreciable excess risk persists for several years. Second, although ethanol is the main responsible for the carcinogenicity of alcoholic beverages, it remains unclear whether different types of alcoholic beverages may have different influences on oral carcinogenesis, and whether spirits are associated to higher risks than beer or wine (Boffetta and Hashibe 2006; Baan et al. 2007). They may contribute to explain some of the exceedingly high rates in countries like Hungary or Slovakia, where, fruit-derived hard spirits are commonly consumed. Acetaldehyde, the main product of ethanol metabolism, has been implicated in the carcinogenicity of alcoholic beverages on the oral mucosa.

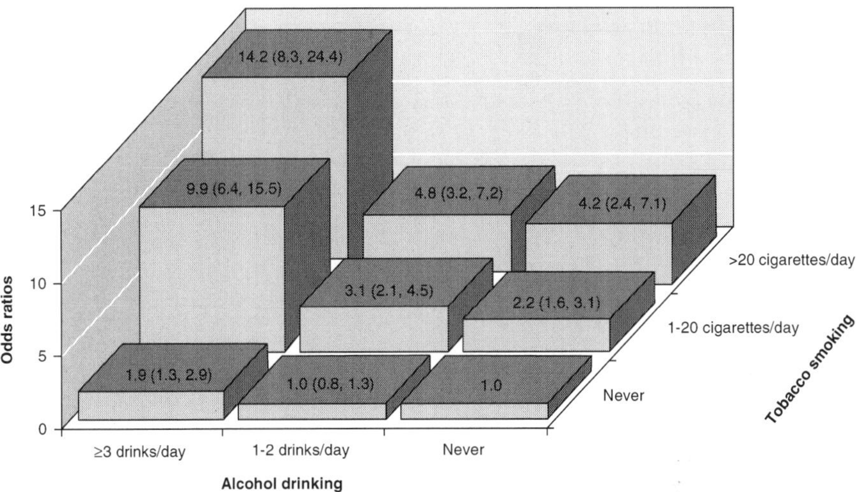

Fig. 4.1 The modifying effect of tobacco on the relation between alcohol drinking and head and neck cancers (modified) (Pelucchi et al. 2011)

Human Papilloma Virus (HPV) DNA is cause of detected in pre-neoplastic and neoplastic lesions of the oral cavity, and it is associated with an over 100-fold excess risk of oropharyngeal cancer and a lesser risk of cancer of the oral cavity (IARC 2007b). In Northern Europe and North America, HPV has become the main risk factor for oral and pharyngeal cancer.

The role of other risk factors on oral cancer incidence and mortality is smaller than that of tobacco or alcohol, and remains largely unquantified. These include dietary and nutritional factors, such as fruit and non starchy vegetable consumption, which have shown a protective effect on oral cavity and pharynx cancer risk (WCRF 2007). Additionally, the role of low socioeconomic status, as well as attained adult height have been reported as risk factors for oral cavity and pharynx cancer, though their effect might be confounded by tobacco/alcohol or childhood nutrition (Conway et al. 2008; Leoncini et al. 2013). Poor oral hygiene and ill-fitting dentures are likely additional risk factors for oral cancer. Several occupations have been sporadically reported to entail an increased risk of oral and pharyngeal cancer. The evidence is somewhat consistent only for employment as a waiter and bartender, probably reflecting an increased consumption of alcohol and tobacco, including involuntary tobacco smoking.

The role of genetic susceptibility in oral carcinogenesis is probably modest. High-risk families have been reported only occasionally. A role is, however, likely for low-penetrance factors, such as increased sensitivity to mutagens and polymorphism of enzymes implicated in the metabolism of alcohol (alcohol dehydrogenase and aldehyde dehydrogenase) (McKay et al. 2011).

4.1.2 Cancer of the Lip

The descriptive epidemiology of lip cancer is made complex by misclassification with lesions from adjacent areas of the skin and the oral mucosa. This neoplasm is rare in most populations and occurs mainly in the lower lip. The main causes are solar radiation, smoking of cigarettes, cigars and pipe, and exposure to polycyclic aromatic hydrocarbons. Consequently, fishermen and farmers were at increased risk. Infection with herpes simplex virus 1 might also play a role.

4.1.3 Cancer of the Nasopharynx

Nasopharyngeal cancer accounts to about 85,000 cases and 52,000 deaths worldwide—(Ferlay et al. 2010b). The geographical distribution of cancer of the nasopharynx shows high-risk areas in southern China, South-East Asia, Northern Africa and the Arctic region (Forman et al. 2013). Migrant populations from these regions are also at increased risk. It is a rare neoplasm in other populations. The male-to-female ratio is in the order of 2–3.

Infection with Epstein–Barr virus (EBV) is causally associated with the development of nasopharyngeal carcinoma, although cofactors, which have not been fully understood, are necessary to the virus to exert its action (Yu and Yuan 2006).

Consumption of Chinese-style salted fish, in particular in childhood, has been associated to increased risk of nasopharyngeal cancer among Cantonese populations from Guangzhou, Hong Kong and the USA, but also in non-Cantonese populations from southern China and Taiwan. Consumption of other types of salted fish might represent a risk factor in South-East Asia and the Arctic. Other preserved foods used as weaning food in different areas of China have also been associated to nasopharyngeal cancer: chung choi (a salted root), salted shrimp paste, salted eggs and preserved fruits. The high rates in northern Africa might be due to consumption of dried mutton, touklia (a spiced mixture of peppers) or harissa (a hot sauce). It is unclear whether the carcinogenic agents in Chinese-style salted fish and other preserved foods are nitrosamines, bacterial mutagens or other genotoxic substances. Low intake of fresh fruits and vegetables has also been associated with increased risk of nasopharyngeal cancer: in high-risk populations, however, low fruit and vegetable intake is often closely associated with high intake of preserved food, making it difficult to separate the effect of the two factors.

Additional suspected risk factors for nasopharyngeal cancer are occupational exposure to formaldehyde and wood dust, exposure to fumes and smoke from burning of organic matter, consumption of Chinese herbal beverages and use of Chinese nasal oil, but these issues remain inconclusive. An association (RR in the order of 3–5) with tobacco smoking has been found in several populations. Chronic inflammatory conditions of the ear, nose and sinuses might act as predisposing factors. Familial aggregation of nasopharyngeal cancer has been shown in China and other high-risk areas: the possible contribution of shared dietary and environmental factors, however, has not been excluded.

Genetic factors play an important role in the etiology of nasopharyngeal carcinoma. In particular, several risk variants in the HLA region have been identified in genomewide studies (Tang et al. 2012).

4.1.4 Cancer of Salivary Glands

Geographical and temporal comparisons of tumours of the salivary glands are complicated by the inclusion of neoplasms with benign or intermediate clinical behaviour in the series of cases. Incidence rates, however, tend to be low, with high rates (in the order of 2–3/100,000) in Hawaii and northern Canada. Men experience higher rates than women, but the ratio rarely exceeds 2 (Forman et al. 2013). Apart from a role of ionizing radiation, the causes of cancer of the salivary glands are unknown. Tobacco smoking does not seem to play a role (Mayne et al. 2006).

4.1.5 Prevention of Oral and Pharyngeal Cancers

Avoidance of tobacco smoking, chewing and snuffing and avoidance of excessive alcohol drinking represent the main preventive measures for cancer of the oral cavity and pharynx. The fact that HPV vaccination will contribute to the prevention of oropharyngeal cancer, is an important argument to extend existing program to boys. It is unclear whether additional benefits might be obtained from increase in fruit and vegetable intake and improvement of oral hygiene. Avoidance of excessive exposure to solar radiation would represent the main preventive approach for lip cancer. In populations at high risk of nasopharyngeal cancer from China and possibly other countries, avoidance of salted fish and other preserved food, in particular as weaning food, should be recommended.

Oral inspection aimed to identify pre-neoplastic lesions is an effective approach for secondary prevention of oral cancer (Sankaranarayanan et al. 2013). The inspection can be performed by medically certified professionals, but also, in particular in high-risk areas from developing countries such as India, by specifically trained health workers.

4.2 Cancer of the Oesophagus

There are two main histological types of oesophageal cancer: squamous cell carcinoma and adenocarcinoma. The former occurs mainly in the upper and middle third of the organ, while adenocarcinoma occurs in the lower third. Squamous Cell

Carcinoma (SqCC) was the predominant type in most human populations, in particular in populations at very high risk. However, recent trend in incidence of adenocarcinoma show considerable rises in North America and Europe, whereas SqCC has been declining in some formerly high incidence and mortality areas, consequently, overall esophageal cancer mortality has been declining in several areas of Europe over the last decade (Bosetti et al. 2008b). In 2012, there were about 450,000 cases and 400,000 deaths from esophageal cancer, worldwide; of these, over 2/3 were in males (Ferlay et al. 2013).

The geographical distribution of oesophageal cancer is characterized by very wide variations within relatively small areas. Very high rates (over 50/100,000) are recorded for both genders in northern Iran and various provinces of eastern China, Shanxi, Henan and Jiangsu, in certain areas of Kazakhstan and among men from Zimbabwe. Intermediate rates in men (10–50/100,000) occur in eastern Africa, southern Brazil, the Caribbean, most of China (with the exception of southern provinces, such as Yunnan, Guizhou, Hunan and Guangxi), regions of Central Asia, Northern India, Southern Europe, as well as in US Blacks (Forman et al. 2013). In all these high-risk areas, SqCC is the predominant histological type. Ethnic factors are suggested by the facts that populations at higher risk in Central Asia are of Turkish or Mongolian origin, and that Blacks in the USA experience in both genders 2–3-fold higher rates than Whites. In men, rates are 2–10-fold higher than in women. In many high-risk areas, a decrease in the incidence of SqCC of the oesophagus has occurred during recent decades. The opposite pattern has been shown in low-risk populations, such as northern Europeans and Whites in the USA. In those countries, the increase was largely accounted for by an increase of adenocarcinoma of the lower oesophagus.

Tobacco smoking is a major risk factor for oesophageal SqCC (Blot et al. 2006). The risk in heavy smokers, relative to non-smokers, is in the order of 5–10. A strong dose–risk relationship has been shown for duration of smoking and average consumption. Quitting smoking substantially reduces the risk: the RR declines within 5 years after quitting, but remains substantially elevated at least 10 years after cessation of smoking, to decline by 40 % thereafter (Bosetti et al. 2006). Thus, cessation of smoking could have an appreciable impact in reducing SqCC esophageal cancer, and represents an obvious priority for prevention and public health purposes. Smoking of black tobacco, high-tar and hand-rolled cigarettes, as well as of pipe, might exert a stronger effect that smoking of other products. Chewing of tobacco-containing products represents an important risk factor in India and southern Africa, but its role has not been confirmed in central Asia. In the latter region, use (smoking and eating) of opium may be (or at least may have been in the past) a reason for the high incidence rates. Snus use has also been related to an excess risk of esophageal cancer, with RR of 3.5 for SqCC a Swedish cohort study (Zendehdel et al. 2008).

Alcohol drinking is the other major risk factor for oesophageal SqCC (Boffetta and Hashibe 2006). In a meta-analysis of 40 case–control and 13 cohort studies, the pooled RRs for esophageal SqCC were 1.38 for light drinking (<12.5 g/day), 2.62 for 12.5–50 g/day, and 5.54 for>50/day. Among never smokers, there was no association for light drinkers, but the RR rose to 3.1 for heavy drinkers. For light drinkers, the association with alcohol was stronger in studies from Asia, indicating a role for genetic factors (including aldehyde dehydrogenase 2-ALDH2-polymorphisms) in Asian populations (Islami et al. 2011). It is unclear whether there are differences in the carcinogenic potency of different alcoholic beverages, but the most common beverage in each population is the most strongly related one. A reduction in the excess risk of oesophageal SqCC is suggested only after several (15–20 years) after quitting. The effect of alcohol is independent from the effect of tobacco, and the interaction between the two exposures fits well a multiplicative model.

Tobacco smoking and alcohol drinking account for 90 % or more of the cases of oesophageal SqCC in Western Europe and North America: this proportion, however, is lower in developing countries, in particular in selected high risk areas of Asia and South America.

Intake of hot maté, a herbal beverage, is an important risk factor for oesophageal SqCC in southern Brazil, Uruguay and northern Argentina. The effect appears to be due to the high temperature: studies from other areas suggest that intake of hot beverages (e.g., hot tea in Iran, Singapore and Japan, hot coffee in Puerto Rico, and hot drinks or soups in Hong Kong) increases the risk of oesophagitis and oesophageal SqCC, although the evidence is less consistent than in the case of maté.

Dietary factors are likely to play a role in the aetiology of oesophageal SqCC. Reduced intake of fresh fruits and vegetables appears to represent a risk factor. A similar effect has been suggested for low intake of fish, for high intake of (red and processed) meat. In general, a dietary pattern rich in foods from animal origin and poor in foods containing vitamins and fiber appears to increase esophageal cancer risk (Bravi et al. 2012). The available data do not, however, allow to establish the potentially preventive role of specific micronutrients from fruits and vegetables, and the results of most chemopreventive trials with retinol, riboflavin, vitamin E, zinc and selenium have failed to show a benefit.

In several areas of China, intake of pickled vegetables has been associated with an increased risk of oesophageal SqCC. The active carcinogens might be mycotoxins or *N*-nitroso compounds. Mycotoxins, including fumonosin B1, have also been detected in moldy corn from high-risk areas in China and southern Africa. In addition, in Japan, eating of bracken fern has been associated with an elevated oesophageal cancer risk. The elucidation of dietary factors implicated in oesophageal carcinogenesis, in particular of the possible role of mycotoxins and *N*-nitroso compounds (including endogenously formed nitrosamines), would represent an important step in the understanding and prevention of this disease. Esophageal cancer is related to ionising radiation, in particular in women irradiated for breast cancer.

Among the other environmental agents suspected to cause oesophageal cancer are infection by HPV and combustion fumes, but these associations are not established.

Patients suffering from Plummer–Vinson syndrome, a sideropenic dysphagia due to deficit of iron, riboflavin and other vitamins, had an increased incidence of hypopharyngeal and oesophageal cancers. Oesophageal cancer risk is also increased among celiac disease patients, possibly because of nutritional deficiencies. Subject with family history of esophageal cancer have or about three excess risk after adjustment for tobacco and alcohol, and the RR rose to over 100-fold in heavy drinker and smokers with positive family history in first degree relatives (Garavello et al. 2005).

A familial aggregation of oesophageal cancer has been occasionally shown, with joint segregation of a gene responsible for keratosis palmaris et plantaris (tylosis). Studies of families without the tylosis gene have not provided evidence of an important role of other high-penetrance genetic susceptibility factors in oesophageal cancer. However, low-penetrance genes, including those encoding for enzymes involved in the metabolism of tobacco and alcohol, may play a role in individual susceptibility to this neoplasm (Lewis and Smith 2005).

4.2.1 Adenocarcinoma

Adenocarcinoma mainly occurs in the lower third of the oesophagus. Its incidence is higher in Western countries, in Whites and in high social class individuals, and has sharply increased in the last decades in most Western countries. In countries such as USA or Scotland, it represents the main type of oesophageal cancer. Barrett's oesophagus, a columnar metaplasia of the epithelium, is strongly associated with the subsequent development of adenocarcinoma. The main risk factor for Barrett's oesophagus and oesophageal adenocarcinoma is persistent reflux oesophagitis.

Adenocarcinoma is related to overweight, obesity, lack of physical activity and gastro-esophageal reflux. In a meta-analysis of 22 studies (Turati et al. 2013b) compared with normal weight individuals, the pooled RR was 1.7 for overweight (BMC 25–30) and 2.3 for obese ones (BMI > 30). The increased prevalence of overweight and inactivity in North America and northern Europe, may partly or largely, explain the increased frequency of adenocarcinoma reported over the last few decades (La Vecchia et al. 2002). Adenocarcinoma of the oesophagus is associated with tobacco smoking and not with alcohol drinking. The pooled RR from a meta-analysis of 33 studies was 1.8 for ever, and 2.36 for current smokers (Tramacere et al. 2011), while a meta-analysis of 20 case–control and 4 cohort studies (Tramacere et al. 2012), reported an overall RR for drinkers versus non drinkers was 1.0–0.9 for moderate and 1.1 for heavy drinkers.

A protective role of high intake of fruits and vegetables and an unfavourable role of intake of salty food has been suggested.

4.2.2 Prevention of Esophageal Cancer

Avoidance of tobacco smoking and elevated alcohol drinking remains the main preventive approach in reducing the burden of oesophageal SqCC in Western populations. Improved diet, in particular increase in consumption of fresh fruits and vegetables, might also contribute to prevention. The incomplete understanding of the role of other factors complicates the elaboration of preventive strategies in many high-risk regions, although a decrease in intake and temperature of hot drink might be important.

Avoidance of tobacco control of obesity, increased physical activity and smoking are the main issues for the prevention of esophageal adenocarcinoma.

Secondary prevention has been attempted in high-risk areas through endoscopy, however, the available evidence does not justify activities at the population level.

4.3 Cancer of the Stomach

Stomach cancer was the fourth most frequent cancer worldwide in 2012, accounting for approximately 950,000 new cases or 7 % of the global cancer burden (Ferlay et al. 2013). More than 70 % of cases occur in developing countries, and half the world total occurs in Eastern Asia (mainly in China). The highest rates are observed in Japan, and more recently in certain counties of China with an age-standardized incidence rate of 169/100,000 in men and 68/100,000 in women (Forman et al. 2013). Low-incidence areas include Eastern and Northern Africa, North America, South-central Asia and Australia (Ferlay et al. 2010b). The rates are approximately twice as high among men as among women and are also 2–3 times higher among groups of low socio-economic status. These were about 720,000 deaths from gastric cancer.

Migrants tend to maintain the high risk of their home country; their offspring tend to acquire a risk closer to their host country. The most striking feature of the epidemiology of stomach cancer is the dramatic decline in its incidence and mortality which has been observed in most countries over the past century. The decline is apparent for both sexes, and has occurred earlier in countries which currently have a low risk. This continuous dramatic decline, as well as the results from migrant studies, suggests a strong environmental influence on the disease.

The reasons for the generalized decline in gastric cancer rates are complex and not completely understood. Almost certainly, these include a more varied and affluent diet and better food conservation, including refrigeration, as well as the control of *Helicobacter pylori* (*H. pylori*) infection. Whether improved diagnosis and treatment has also played some role on the favorable trends in gastric cancer, particularly over most recent calendar periods, however, remains open to question.

Several intervention trials have also been conducted involving nutrient supplements and stomach cancer. In one of these trials, which was conducted in a Chinese population known to be micronutrient deficient, a combination supplement of β-carotene, vitamin E and selenium did result in a small reduction in the risk of stomach cancer (Blot 1997), but recent findings on the issue on other, better nourished populations, are largely negative (Plummer et al. 2007; WCRF 2007).

Regarding beverages, no evidence has been found that black tea, coffee or alcohol influence the risk of stomach cancer (Tramacere et al. 2012). Throughout the world there is a strong and consistent correlation between consumption of salt and salted foods and stomach cancer incidence. A joint report from the World Cancer Research Fund and the American Institute for Cancer Research (WCRF/AICR) concluded that there is 'probable evidence' that high consumption of non-starchy vegetables and fruits decreases the risk of gastric cancer, while salt and salted foods are likely to increase the risk (WCRF 2007). The relationship is also biologically plausible given that salt may lead to damage of the protective mucosal layer of the stomach. Other methods of food preservation, including curing and smoking foods, have also been associated with stomach cancer, although the evidence is not consistent.

An increased risk of gastric cancer is associated with *H. pylori* infection. The biological plausibility of a causal association is also supported by a strong association between *H. pylori* and precancerous lesions, including chronic and atrophic gastritis and dysplasia. Given that the prevalence of infection is very high, especially in developing counties and among older cohorts, *H. pylori* can explain over 50 % of all new cases of gastric cancer that occur, or over 5 % of all cancer cases globally (Parkin 2006). The extent to which different strains of *H. pylori*, for example those containing the *cagA* gene, have different carcinogenic potential, however, is unclear (Kato et al. 2007; Boccia and La Vecchia 2013).

Another important cause of stomach cancer is tobacco smoking. Smokers have a 50–60 % increased risk of stomach cancer, as compared to non-smokers. This relationship would indicate that smoking is responsible for approximately 10 % of all cases (IARC 2004; Ladeiras-Lopes et al. 2008).

Gastric cancer risk is elevated 2–3-fold in subjects with family history of the disease (La Vecchia et al. 1992). Several genes involved in the protection of gastric mucosa against damaging agents, in inflammatory response, in detoxification of carcinogens, in the synthesis and repair of DNA, in folate metabolism, in the regulation of gene expression and in cell adhesion and the cell cycle have been considered in relation to gastric cancer risk. These include the polymorphic glutathione-S-transferase (GSTM1) gene, GSTT1 deficiency, the combination of GSTT1 and GSTM1 deficiency, and methylenetetrahydrofolate reductase (MTHFR) C677T polymorphism, particularly in individuals reporting low folate intake (Boccia et al. 2006; Boccia and La Vecchia 2013).

4.3.1 Prevention of Stomach Cancer

Primary prevention of stomach cancer by dietary means is feasible by encouraging high-risk populations to decrease consumption of cured meats and salt preserved foods. Prevention may also be feasible through eradication of *H. pylori* infection, particularly in childhood and adolescence, by avoiding mother to child transmission. Screening and early detection of stomach cancer have been developed in Japan with use of X-ray photofluorography to identify possible early lesions, followed by gastroscopy. Screen-detected cases are more likely to be early stage localized disease and are likely to have a greater survival than other cases. Screening and early detection is not considered cost-effective in populations outside high-incidence areas.

4.4 Cancer of the Intestines

Cancer of the intestine is a major human neoplasm, in particular among non-smokers and its rates are high in particular in high-income countries. Most cancers of the intestine occur in the large intestine, while cancer of the small intestine is rare. Of colorectal cancers, approximately two-thirds originate from the colon and one-third from the rectum and the rectosigmoid junction. Most cancers of the intestine are of adenocarcinoma type, that is, originate from the glandular cells. Other histological types include carcinoids, sarcomas and lymphomas.

When taken together, cancers of the colon and rectum accounted in 2012 for about 1,360,000 new cases and 700,000 deaths worldwide (Ferlay et al. 2013). They represent the third most frequent malignant disease in terms of incidence and the fourth for mortality.

4.4.1 Cancer of the Small Intestine

Age-standardized incidence rates of small intestinal cancer are in most populations below 2/100,000 persons in both genders. The highest rates (in the order of 3/100,000) are registered among Blacks in the USA and in Western Europe (Forman et al. 2013). The neoplasm is more common in men than in women, with a ratio in the order of 1.5–3. Its occurrence is correlated with the incidence of colon cancer but not stomach cancer.

Adenocarcinomas account for approximately 50 % of neoplasms of the small intestine. They originate mainly in the duodenum and proximal jejunum and are preceded by formation of adenoma. Various hereditary syndromes such as familial adenomatous polyposis and Peutz-Jeghers syndrome, are characterized by multiple hamartomatous adenomas of the small intestine and, to a less extent, of the colon: these patients carry an increased risk of adenocarcinoma of the small intestine. Similarly, patients with Crohn's disease have a tenfold increased risk of small intestine adenocarcinoma (Beebe-Dimer and Schottenfeld 2006). Overweight/obesity is the only known modifiable risk factor of small intestine adenocarcinoma.

Malignant lymphomas represent about one-fourth of neoplasms of the small intestine: they are mainly of diffuse histiocytic type. Patients with acquired immunodeficiency syndrome and celiac sprue are at increased risk of small cell lymphomas. Carcinoid tumours, which originate from the enteroendocrine (argentaffin) cells, are another important histological type. Limited data are available on the risk factors for this type of neoplasm.

The evidence for a role of environmental factors, such as tobacco smoking, alcohol and diet, in the genesis of small intestine neoplasms is at present inconclusive.

4.4.2 Colon Cancer

The highest rates of colon cancer (around or above 30/100,000 in men and 25/100,000 in women) are recorded in Oceania, the USA (in particular among Blacks) and Western Europe. Rates in low- and medium-income countries are lower (5–15/100,000), although they are increasing (Forman et al. 2013). In most populations, rates are higher in men than in women, with a ratio in the order of 1.5; however, given the predominance of women at older ages, the number of cases is similar in the two genders. A small increase in the incidence of colon cancer has been observed during the last decades in most populations, but mortality has been declining in North America and Western Europe over the last two decades (Fernandez et al. 2005).

Studies of migrant populations have shown that the risk of colon cancer approaches that of the country of adoption within one generation; the incidence is higher in urban than in rural populations.

The predominant histological type of malignant neoplasms of the colon is adenocarcinoma. This neoplasm is usually preceded by a polyp, or adenoma, less frequently by a small area of flat mucosa exhibiting various grades of dysplasia. The malignant potential of an adenoma is increased by a surface diameter greater than 1 cm, by villous (rather than tubular) organization and by severe cellular dysplasia. Carriers of one adenoma larger than 1 cm have a 2–4 times increased risk of developing colon cancer; this risk is further doubled in carriers of multiple adenomas. On a geographical basis, the prevalence of adenomas detected during colonoscopy closely parallels the incidence of colon cancer.

Migrant studies suggest that dietary factors are responsible for a substantial proportion of colorectal cancer; however, recent evidence from perspective studies provides only limited evidence in favour of a role of specific foods and nutrients (WCRF 2007). The strongest evidence concerns an increased risk for high intake of meat and of smoked, salted or processed foods. A protective role of high intake of fruits and vegetables has been reported, but is still open to discussion. The role of micronutrients, including in particular Vitamin D, remains unclear, although there is growing evidence of a protective effect of calcium (Chan and Giovannucci 2010).

Increased use of aspirin and other anti-inflammatory drugs is likely to have reduced the incidence of colorectal cancer (Bosetti et al. 2012d). Hormone therapy in menopause and other female hormones, including OC, have been inversely related to colon cancer risks, and hence may also play some protective role. In addition life-style factors, such as excessive alcohol consumption, lack of physical activity, and overweight/obesity increase the risk of the disease.

Several studies have associated tobacco smoking with an increased risk of colonic adenoma. For colon cancer, a modest increased risk following prolonged heavy smoking has been shown in some of the largest prospective studies (IARC 2004).

Patients with ulcerative colitis and Crohn's disease are at increased risk of colon cancer. The overall RR has been estimated in the range of 5–20, and it is higher for young age at diagnosis, severity of the disease, and presence of dysplasia. The contribution of shared genetic and environmental factors in the genesis of the two inflammatory conditions and of colon cancer is not known. Diabetes and cholecystectomy have been associated with a moderate (1.5–2-fold) increased risk of colon cancer, possibly due to continuous secretion of bile. Patients with one cancer of the colon have a double risk to develop a second primary tumour in the colon or rectum, and the relative risk is greater for early age at first diagnosis. In women, an association has been shown also with cancers of the endometrium, ovary and breast, possibly due to shared hormonal or dietary factors.

There are several rare hereditary conditions that are characterized by a very high incidence of colon cancer. Familial adenomatous polyposis, due to inherited or de novo mutation in the adenomatous polyposis colon gene on chromosome 5, is characterized by a very high number of colonic adenomas and a cumulative incidence of colon or rectal cancer close to 100 % by age 55. Other, rarer, diseases characterized by colonic polyposis, among other features, are Gardner's syndrome, Turcot syndrome and juvenile polyposis. All these hereditary conditions, although very serious for the affected patients, account for no more than 1 % of colon cancers in the general population.

Two syndromes characterized by hereditary non-polyposis colon cancer, that is, with increased familial risk of colon cancer in the absence of adenomas, have been described. Lynch syndrome I is characterized by increased risk of cancer of the proximal (right) colon, and is due to inherited mutation in one of two genes involved in DNA repair. Patients of Lynch syndrome II have also an increased risk of extracolonic neoplasms, mainly of the endometrium and the breast. As a whole, hereditary non-polyposis colon cancer may account for a sizeable proportion of cases of colon cancer in Western populations. In addition to these hereditary conditions, first-degree relatives of colon cancer patients have a 2–3-fold increased risk of developing a cancer of the colon or the rectum. Genomewide association studies have identified risk variants in several genes, including those involved in DNA repair and cell cycle control (Peters et al. 2013).

4.4.3 Cancer of the Rectum

The distribution of cancer of the rectum, including the rectosigmoid junction and the anus, parallels the distribution of colon cancer: the highest rates are recorded in Europe and Japan and are in the order of 35/100,000 in men and 10/100,000 in women (Parkin et al. 2002). In most populations, incidence rates have been stable in recent decades. The male-to-female ratio is close to 2. The colon/rectum cancer incidence ratio is below 1 in India and East Asia, while it is higher than 2.5 in Italy, South America and US Blacks.

Most biological and epidemiological features of rectal cancer resemble those described for colon cancer, including the pre-neoplastic role of adenomas and non-polypoid dysplastic mucosa, the presence of familial syndromes, the increased risk among patients with chronic inflammatory bowel diseases, and the likely protective role of dietary factors and physical activity. In addition, several studies have provided evidence, although not fully consistent, of an association between elevated intake of alcohol, and increased risk of colorectal adenoma and adenocarcinoma (Baan et al. 2007).

Moreover, total mesorectal excision and adjuvant radiotherapy have provided excellent local tumour control and improved survival for rectal cancer.

4.4.4 Cancer of the Anus

The incidence of cancer of the anus is, in most male populations, between 0.5 and 1.5/100,000. This neoplasm may occur either in the anal canal or in the perianal region; the predominant histological types are squamous cell carcinoma and transitional cell carcinoma. Women have a higher incidence of cancer of the anus, in particular of the canal, than men.

The epidemiological features of the disease resemble those of sexually transmitted diseases, with an increased incidence among never married persons, men with homosexual preference and persons with an increased number of sexual partners. The disease has also been associated with previous or subsequent history of cancers of the uterine cervix, vagina, vulva and penis (Frisch and Melbye 2006).

Chronic infection with HPV, in particular types 16 and 18, is the main known risk factor for anal squamous cell carcinoma. HPV DNA has been detected both in a high proportion of carcinomas and anal intraepithelial neoplasias, the precursor lesions of invasive cancer.

4.4.5 Prevention of Intestinal Cancers

Increased physical activity and avoidance of overweight and obesity are the main tools for the primary prevention of colorectal cancer. Chemopreventive strategies cannot be recommended at present. Control of HPV infection, possibly via vaccination in new generations, would represent the main preventive measure for anal cancer.

Surveillance via flexible colonoscopy, involving removal of adenomas, is a secondary preventive measure. An additional approach consists in the detection of fecal occult blood. The method suffers from low specificity and, to a lesser extent, low sensitivity, in particular in the ability to detect adenomas. However, trials have shown a reduced mortality from colorectal cancer after annual test, although this is achieved at a high cost due to an elevated number of false positive cases. Current recommendations for individuals aged 50 and over include either annual faecal occult blood testing or once colonoscopy (Smith et al. 2013). The WHO has endorsed in 2011 the recommendations of the Council of The European Union of 2003, that advice for population-based screening of colorectal cancer, though the cost-effectiveness remains somewhat contested (Sigurdsson et al. 2013).

4.5 Cancer of the Liver and Biliary Tract

Worldwide, about 780,000 cases of liver cancer were registered in 2012, with 750,000 deaths. Over two-third of cases are in men (Ferlay et al. 2013).

The epidemiology of liver cancer is made complex by the large number of secondary tumours, which are difficult to separate from primary liver cancers without histological verification. The most common histological type of liver malignant neoplasm is Hepatocellular Carcinoma (HCC). Other forms include: (1) childhood hepatoblastoma, and (2) adult cholangiocarcinoma (originating from the intrahepatic biliary ducts) and (3) angiosarcoma (from the intrahepatic blood vessels). Cancers of the extrahepatic biliary ducts are of the adenocarcinoma type. Most HCC originate from cirrhotic tissue.

The incidence of liver cancer is high in all low-resource regions of the world, with the exception of Northern Africa and Western Asia. The highest rates (above 40/100,000 in men and above 10/100,000 in women) are recorded in Thailand, Korea and certain parts of China. In most high-resource countries, age-standardized rates are below 10/100,000 in men and 3/100,000 in women. Intermediate rates (10–20/100,000 in men) are observed in areas of Southern and Central Europe (Forman et al. 2013). Rates are 2–3-folds higher in men than women, and the difference is stronger in high-incidence than in low-incidence areas. The estimated worldwide number of new cases of liver cancer in 2008 is 750,000, of which more than 80 % are from developing countries (54 % from China alone) (Ferlay et al. 2010b). Given the poor survival from this disease, the estimated number of deaths is similar to that of new cases (695,000): liver cancer is the second most frequent cause of neoplastic death in low-resource countries.

Incidence and mortality from primary liver cancer have been rising among middle age men in the USA (El-Serag 2004), but not consistently in Europe, over the last few decades.

Incidence rates of biliary tract cancer, including gallbladder, are high (above 3/100,000 in men and above 5/100,000 in women) in Central Europe, South America, Northern India, Japan, Korea and Western Asia. In the USA, rates are higher among people of American-Indian, Hispanic and Japanese origin than in other groups. Most of the geographical variation is accounted for by cancer of the gallbladder, which represents the majority of biliary tract cancers. Rates of gallbladder cancer in women are generally higher than in men, while other biliary tract cancers are slightly more frequent in men.

4.5.1 Hepatocellular Carcinoma

Chronic infections with Hepatitis B Virus (HBV) and Hepatitis B Virus (HCV) are the main causes of HCC. The risk increases with early age at infection (in high-risk countries, most HBV infections occur perinatally or in early childhood), and the presence of liver cirrhosis is a pathogenic step. HBV is the main agent in China,

South-East Asia and Africa, while HCV is the predominant virus in Japan, North America and Southern Europe. The most frequent routes of HCV transmission are parenteral HCC and sexual, while perinatal infection is rare. The estimated risk of developing HCC among infected subjects, relative to uninfected, ranged between 10 and 50 in different studies. On a global scale, the fraction of liver cancer cases attributable to HBV is 54 %, the one attributable to HCV is 31 % (Parkin 2006).

Ecological studies have shown that the incidence of HCC correlates not only with HBV and HCV infection, but also with contamination of foodstuff with aflatoxins, a group of mycotoxins produced by the fungi *Aspergillus flavus* and *Aspergillus parasiticus*, which cause liver cancer in many species of experimental animals. Contamination originates mainly from improper storage of cereals, peanuts and other vegetables and is prevalent in particular in Africa, South-East Asia and China. Prospective studies have shown a strong association between biological markers of aflatoxin exposure in serum or urine and risk of subsequent liver cancer; the carcinogenic effect of aflatoxins, in particular of aflatoxin B_1, was shown to be independent from—and to interact with—that exerted by HBV infection (London and McGlynn 2006).

Alcohol intake increases the risk of HCC. The most likely mechanism is through development of cirrhosis, although alternative mechanisms such as alteration in activation and detoxification of carcinogens may also play a role. Alcoholic cirrhosis is probably the most important risk factors for HCC in populations with low prevalence of HBV and HCV infection and low exposure to aflatoxins, such as North America and Northern Europe (La Vecchia 2007). The association between tobacco smoking and HCC is now established, with a RR of the order of 1.5–2 (Gandini et al. 2008).

Use of oral contraceptives (OC) greatly increases the risk of liver adenomas, and is associated with the risk of HCC, although the absolute risk is likely to be small (IARC 2007b; Cibula et al. 2010). Case reports have associated use of anabolic steroids with development of liver cancer, but the evidence is not conclusive. An increase in iron storage in the body is a likely cause of HCC: the evidence comes from studies of patients with hemochromatosis or other disorders of iron metabolism. The effect of iron overload seems to be independent from development of cirrhosis and may interact with HBV infection.

Diabetes is also related to an excess risk of HCC, and the increased prevalence of overweight and obesity, and consequently of diabetes, in several populations may have had some role in recent unfavourable trends of HCC in North America and other areas of the world. Combined exposure to overweight at diabetes led to a RR of HCC of 4.75, after allowance for hepatitis, alcohol and other recognised possible confounding factors (Turati et al. 2013b).

The excess risk of liver cancer associated with overweight/obesity and diabetes has been related to the development of non-alcoholic fatty liver disease (NAFLD) (Sanyal et al. 2010). NAFLD is characterised by excess fat accumulation in the liver, and ranges from isolated hepatic steatosis to non-alcoholic steatohepatitis (NASH), the more aggressive form of fatty liver disease, which can progress to cirrhosis and HCC. However, NAFLD/NASH increases HCC risk even in the absence of cirrhosis (Turati et al. 2013a) (Fig. 4.2).

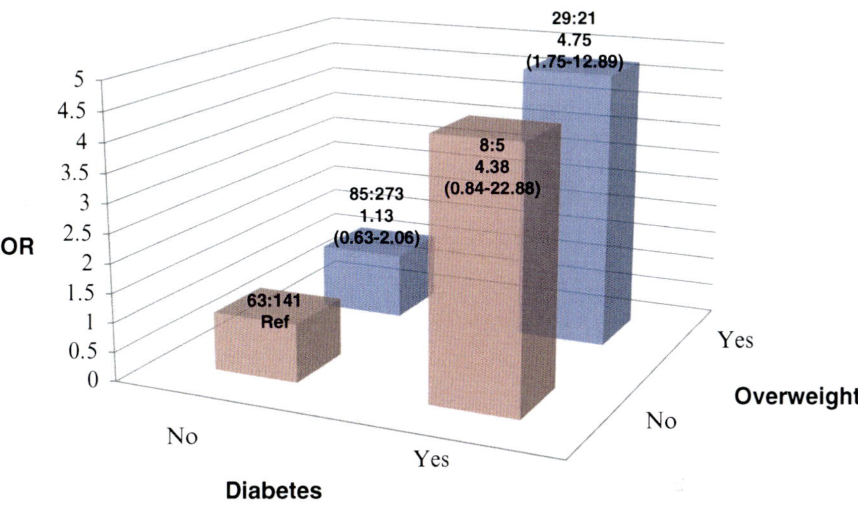

Fig. 4.2 Combined effect of overweight and diabetes on HCC risk from (Turati et al. 2013a)

4.5.2 *Other Types of Primary Liver Cancer*

Infestation with the liver flukes, *Opistorchis viverrini* and *Clonorchis sinensis*, is the main known cause of this form of cholangiocarcinoma that is rare in most populations but relatively frequent in infested areas in South-East Asia. Infection occurs via consumption of improperly cooked fish. Exposure to thorotrast, a contrast medium containing radioactive thorium used for angiography in Europe and Japan during 1930–1955, resulted in an increase of cholangiocarcinoma and of liver angiosarcoma. Workers exposed to vinyl chloride, a monomer used in the chemical industry for production of the plastic polymer, polyvinyl chloride, experience an increased risk of angiosarcoma. The identification of clusters of cases of liver angiosarcoma in these workers has led to a drastic reduction in occupational exposure to vinyl chloride.

4.5.3 *Cancer of Extrahepatic Biliary Ducts*

The main known risk factor for cancer of the gallbladder is presence of gallstones. The RR is in the order of 3, and it is higher in patients with large (>3 cm in diameter) rather than small (<1 cm) stones. In Western populations, most gallstones are formed by cholesterol, and their formation is associated with hypersecretion and saturation of cholesterol in the bile. The possible causes of cholesterol saturation (obesity, multiple pregnancies and other hormonal factors) are also associated with increased risk of gallbladder cancer. An additional role of gallbladder hypomotility in stone formation is likely. In Asia, the main types of gallstone are formed by bilirubin salts and have as risk factor bacterial infection of the biliary system: their association with gallbladder cancer, however, is not clear (Hsing et al. 2006). The increased rate of cholecystectomy in many high resource countries is probably responsible for the temporal decreasing trend of gallbladder cancer (Randi et al. 2006).

Other suspected risk factors for gallbladder cancer include chronic inflammation, biliary stasis and infection, in particular status of chronic typhoid and paratyphoid carrier, history of gastric resection, reproductive history resulting in increased exposure to endogenous oestrogens and progesterone, obesity and, possibly, increased energy intake. It is likely that these factors act through gallstone formation, although the available data do not allow a conclusion with respect to their possible role in gallbladder carcinogenesis.

Fewer data are available on risk factors for cancer of extrahepatic biliary ducts. Infestation with the liver flukes causing intrahepatic cholangiocarcinoma, and history of ulcerative colitis are established risk factors but explain only a small proportion of these cancers. Tobacco smoking and diabetes have been suggested as additional causes. The incidence of gallbladder cancer has increase in Europe during the last two decades (Jepsen et al. 2007).

Genetic factors are likely to play a role in biliary tract cancer. Patients with hereditary cancer-prone conditions, such as ataxia-telangiectasia and hereditary non-polyposis colon cancer, have an increased risk of biliary tract cancer. Furthermore, a familial aggregation has been shown in population-based studies, which might be due to familial predisposition to gallstone formation.

4.5.4 Prevention of Liver Cancer and Biliary Tract Cancers

The strong role in liver carcinogenesis of infection with HBV, a virus for which effective and cheap vaccines are available, indicates that a large proportion of liver cancers are preventable. In high-prevalence areas, HBV vaccination should be introduced in the perinatal period. In the last decades, many countries from Asia, Southern Europe and, to a lesser extent, Africa have expanded the national childhood vaccination programme to include HBV. A similar primary preventive approach is not available for HCV. Control of transmissions is however feasible and medical treatment of carriers with interferon might represent an alternative approach (which is also available for HBV carriers).

Control of aflatoxin contamination of foodstuffs represents another important preventive measure. While this is easily achieved in high-income countries, its implementation is limited by economic and logistic factors in many high-prevalence regions. Control of tobacco smoking and excessive alcohol drinking represents additional primary preventive measures.

Ultrasound has been proposed as screening method for liver cancer, but its effectiveness has not been proven. In general, population-based studies are currently available showing a decreased mortality from liver cancer in screened populations.

Cholecystectomy is an obvious mean to prevent gallbladder cancer. The removal of the gallbladder in asymptomatic patients, however, is not justified, with the possible exception of high-risk circumstances such as large stones and calcified gallbladder.

4.6 Cancer of the Pancreas

The great majority of malignant neoplasms of the pancreas are adenocarcinomas which originate from the exocrine portion secreting digestive enzymes. Rare pancreatic neoplasms include tumours (of uncertain clinical behaviour) of the endocrine portion, which secretes insulin and glucagon, as well as lymphomas and sarcomas.

There are geographical and temporal variations in the sensitivity and specificity of clinical diagnosis and in the proportion of histological verification of pancreatic cancer cases. Even when comparing populations living in the same place at the same time (e.g., different social classes or age groups), differential access to health care might affect incidence and mortality data.

The highest rates are recorded among Blacks in the USA (12–15/100,000 in men and 8–10/100,000 in women) and among indigenous populations in Oceania. The lowest rates, which may suffer from under-diagnosis, are recorded in India, and Northern and Central Africa (below 2/100,000 in men and 1/100,000 in women). In the USA, rates are about 30–50 % higher in Blacks as compared to Whites living in the same areas (Forman et al. 2013). The disease accounts for an estimated 340,000 new cases in 2012, 60 % of which occurred in high-income countries (Ferlay et al. 2013). Given the very poor survival, mortality rates closely parallel incidence rates. Rates are about 50 % higher in men than in women. An increase in incidence and mortality has taken place since the 1970s, in particular in Europe, that can be attributed in part to diagnostic improvements. However, incidence and mortality have levelled off and declined over recent years in Western Europe and North America (Bosetti et al. 2012a).

Urban populations have higher rates than rural ones, but this may again reflect differences in quality of diagnosis. Migrant studies suggest that first-generation migrants from low- to high-risk areas experience, after 15 or 20 years, rates that are even higher than those of the country of migration, suggesting an important role of environmental exposures occurring late in life (Anderson et al. 2006).

The best known risk factor for pancreatic cancer is tobacco smoking. The risk in smokers is about twofold higher than that in non-smokers (Gandini et al. 2008), and a dose–response relationship and a favourable effect of quitting smoking have been shown in many populations. The proportion of cases of pancreatic cancer attributable to tobacco smoking has been estimated to be 15–20 % (Bosetti et al. 2012b). Some of the features of the descriptive epidemiology of pancreatic cancer (that is, a high incidence among Blacks in the USA as compared to a low incidence in Africa, and a higher risk among men and urban residents) can be explained by differences in smoking habits. Use of smokeless tobacco products is likely to increase the risk of the disease (Boffetta et al. 2008).

Nutritional and dietary factors have been suggested as related to pancreatic cancer, including obesity and low physical activity, high intake of (saturated) fats and low intake of vegetables and fruit (WCRF 2007). The issue of nutrition, diet and pancreatic cancer remains however largely undefined.

Early reports of an association between coffee consumption and pancreatic cancer risk have not been confirmed by larger, more recent investigations. A positive association between heavy alcohol drinking and pancreatic cancer has been observed in epidemiologic studies (Tramacere et al. 2010).

Several medical conditions have been studied with respect to their association with subsequent risk of pancreatic cancer. History of pancreatitis increases the risk more than tenfold, with little difference between the alcoholic and non-alcoholic forms of the disease. An increased risk has also been shown in several studies of diabetic patients; the RR is likely to fall in the range 1.5–2 and is higher in the short term after diagnosis of diabetes. Gastrectomy patients are at 3–5-fold increased risk of pancreatic cancer; the association does not appear to be confounded by tobacco smoking.

A familial history of cancer of the pancreas is present is 8–10 % of patients, suggesting a possible role for genetic factors. Specific hereditary conditions carrying an increased risk of pancreatic cancer include the Li–Fraumeni syndrome, and hereditary non-polyposis colon cancer. Genes associated with pancreatic cancer include high-penetrance genes such as BRCA1 and PALB2, and common variants entailing a modest risk, such as those in at the ABO blood group locus (Rizzato et al. 2013).

There is no effective cure for pancreatic cancer, with the exception of surgery for a small number of patients. Screening methods are being explored but are not currently available. Primary prevention is the only available tool for this disease: avoidance of smoking is the major practicable day for reducing the number of cases. Control of obesity is another potential preventive measure.

4.7 Cancer of the Respiratory Tract

4.7.1 Cancer of the Nasal Cavity and the Paranasal Sinuses

The incidence of cancer of the nasal cavity and paranasal sinuses (sinonasal cancer) is low in most populations (<1/100,000 in men and <0.5/100,000 in women). Higher rates are recorded in Japan and certain parts of China and India. In Europe, North America and Japan, squamous cell carcinoma is the main histological type, followed by adenocarcinoma, and 30–40 % of the cancers originate from the maxillary sinus. In other countries, other forms of sinonasal cancer are important, such as Burkitt's lymphoma of the maxillary or ethmoid sinus in Eastern Africa (Forman et al. 2013). Time trends have shown in most populations a stable incidence or a decline in recent decades.

Known risk factors of sinonasal cancer include occupational exposure to wood dust, in particular to dust of hard woods such as beech and oak: the increase in risk (in the order of 5–50-fold) is strongest for adenocarcinoma and for cancers originating from the sinuses. It is unclear whether dust from soft woods such as pine and spruce increases the risk. An increased risk of sinonasal adenocarcinoma has been shown among workers exposed to leather dust, in particular in shoe manufacturing, and among workers in nickel refining and chromate pigment manufacture, but not among workers exposed to these metals in other processes, such as plating and welding. In addition, exposure to mineral oils, formaldehyde, textile dust and radium-226 might increase the risk of this cancer, but the issue remains unresolved (Littman and Vaughan 2006).

Tobacco smoking is an additional risk factor of sinonasal cancer, and in particular squamous cell carcinoma, with RR in the range 2–5. Presence of recurrent polyps represents an additional risk factor. Suggestive evidence is available for an etiologic role of involuntary tobacco smoking, snuff use, and infection with EBV and HPV.

4.7.2 Cancer of the Larynx

More than 90 % of cancers of the larynx are squamous cell carcinomas, and the majority originate from the supraglottic and glottic regions of the organs. The incidence in men is high (10/100,000 or more) in Southern and Central Europe, and South America, while the lowest rates (<1/100,000) are recorded in South-East Asia and Central Africa. The incidence in women is below 1/100,000 in most populations (Forman et al. 2013). In the US, Black have 50–70 % higher incidence than Whites. In most high-income countries rates have declined in men over the last two decades. An estimated 160,000 new cases occurred worldwide in 2008, of which 140,000 among men (Ferlay et al. 2013). The estimated global number of deaths was 84,000.

Up to 80 % of cases of laryngeal cancer in high-income countries are attributable to tobacco smoking, alcohol drinking and the interaction between the two factors (Olshan 2006). The effect of tobacco, with risks in smokers in the order of 10 relative to non-smokers, seems to be stronger for glottic than supraglottic neoplasms. Studies in several populations have shown a dose–response relationship and a beneficial effect of quitting smoking. Smoking black-tobacco cigarettes entails a stronger risk than smoking blond-tobacco cigarettes. Studies from India have also reported an effect of chewing tobacco-containing products. The effect of alcohol is stronger for supraglottic tumours than for tumours at other sites: it is not clear, however, whether different alcoholic beverages exert a different carcinogenic effect.

There are suggestions of a protective effect exerted by high intake of fruits and vegetables, although the evidence is not conclusive and the date regarding specific micronutrients, such as carotenoids and vitamin C, are inadequate (WCRF 2007). Data concerning a possible effect of other foods are not consistent.

Occupational exposure to mists of strong inorganic acids, in particular of sulfuric acid, and to asbestos fibres are suspected causes of laryngeal cancer. A possible effect has been suggested for other occupational exposures, including nickel and ionizing radiation, but the evidence is not conclusive.

An etiological role of HPV infection has been suggested by the association of this infection with oropharyngeal cancer and by the observation that laryngeal papillomatosis, a condition characterized by multiple benign papillomas caused by infection with HPV types 6 and 11, entails an increased risk of laryngeal cancer. However, studies aimed at assessing the presence of HPV DNA have provided contrasting results (Li et al. 2013).

There are no recognised of strong genetic factors in laryngeal carcinogenesis; however, polymorphism for enzymes implicated in the metabolism of alcohol might represent susceptibility factors (McKay et al. 2011).

Survival from laryngeal cancer is relatively common (5-year survival rates are in the order of 65 % in developed countries and 40 % in developing countries). These patients are at very high risk of developing a second primary tumour in the oral cavity, pharynx and lung. While shared risk factors are likely to play an important role, it is plausible that host factors are also partially responsible.

Control of tobacco smoking and excessive alcohol drinking, possibly together with an increased intake of fruits and vegetables, would prevent the majority of cases of laryngeal cancer in most populations. Control of exposure to suspected occupational carcinogens is an additional potential preventive measure for exposed workers. No screening methods are currently available for laryngeal cancer.

4.7.3 Lung Cancer

Lung cancer was a rare disease until the beginning of the twentieth century. Since then, its occurrence has increased rapidly and this neoplasm has become the most frequent malignant neoplasm among men in most countries, and represents the most important cause of cancer death worldwide. It accounts for an estimated 1,250,000 new cases and 1,100,000 deaths each year among men and 580,000 cases and 500,000 deaths among women (Ferlay et al. 2013). Survival from lung cancer is poor (around 10 % at 5 years).

The geographical and temporal patterns of lung cancer incidence are to a large extent determined by consumption of tobacco. An increase in tobacco consumption is paralleled some decades later by an increase in the incidence of lung cancer; similarly, a decrease in consumption is followed by a decrease in incidence.

The highest incidence rates in men (>80/100,000) are recorded among Blacks from the United States and in some Central and Eastern-European countries

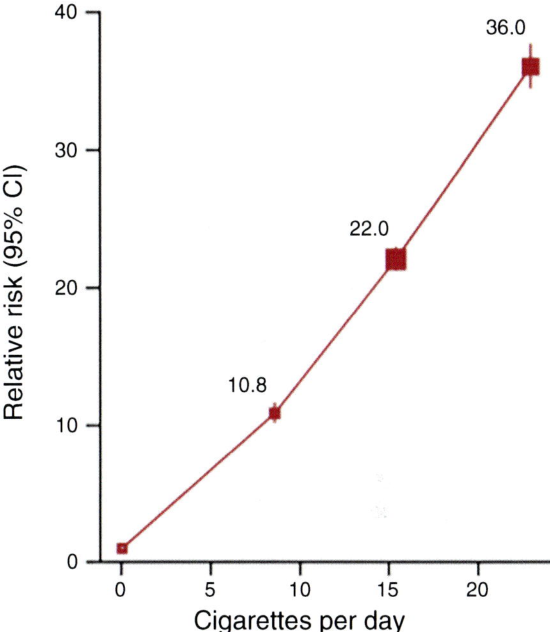

Fig. 4.3 Relative risk of lung cancer according to number of cigarette smoked in the Millon Women Study (Pirie et al. 2013)

(Forman et al. 2013). Rates are declining among US White men and among men in United Kingdom and Northern Europe. The lowest incidence rates are reported from Africa and Southern Asia.

Rates in women are high (>30/100,000) in the USA, Canada, Northern Europe and parts of China, and low (<10/100,000) in and Spain and Arabic countries, in which the prevalence of smoking in women increased only recently.

The main histological types of lung cancer are squamous cell carcinoma, small cell carcinoma, adenocarcinoma, and large cell carcinoma. Over the last decades, the proportion of squamous cell carcinomas, which used to be the predominant type, has decreased and an increase of adenocarcinomas has taken place in both genders. Despite some minor differences, the main risk factors for lung cancer affect all histological types.

A carcinogenic effect of tobacco smoke on the lung has been demonstrated in the 1950s and has been recognized by public health and regulatory authorities since the mid 1960s (IARC 2004). The risk of lung cancer among smokers relative to the risk among never-smokers is in the order of over 20-fold. In the UK million women study, the RRs of lung cancer were 10.5 for current smokers of 10 cigarettes per day, 22.0 for 15, and 36.0 for ≥20 cigarettes per day (Fig. 4.3) (Pirie et al. 2013). Thus, even moderate smokers have a substantial excess lung cancer mortality. This overall risk reflects the contribution of the different aspects of tobacco smoking: average consumption, duration of smoking, time since quitting, age at start, type of tobacco product and inhalation pattern, with duration being the dominant factor. As compared to continuous smokers, the excess risk levelly off in ex-smokers after quitting, but a small excess risk is likely to persist in long-term quitters throughout life. In the United Kingdom, the cumulative risk of lung cancer of a continuous smoker is 16 % and it is reduced to 10 %, 6 %, 3 % and 2 % among those who stopped at age 60, 50, 40 and 30, respectively (Peto et al. 2000). Smokers of black (air-cured) tobacco cigarettes are at higher risk of lung cancer than smokers of blond (flue-cured) tobacco cigarettes. A causal association with lung cancer has been shown also for consumption of cigars, cigarillos, pipe, bidis, water pipe and other smoking tobacco products.

An association has been shown in many studies between exposure to involuntary smoking and lung cancer risk in non-smokers. The magnitude of the excess risk among non-smokers exposed to involuntary smoking is in the order 20 % (IARC 2004).

There is limited evidence that a diet rich in vegetables and fruits exerts a protective effect against lung cancer (WCRF 2007). Despite the many studies of intake of other foods, such as cereals, pulses, meat, eggs, milk and dairy products, the evidence is inadequate to allow a judgement regarding the evidence of a carcinogenic or a protective effect.

Intervention trials of β-carotene supplementation have shown an increase in the incidence of lung cancer in the treated groups; it is unclear whether high dietary exposure to β-carotene entails a risk (Albanes et al. 1996).

There is inadequate evidence of an increase in the risk of lung cancer from heavy alcohol drinking, independent from tobacco smoking (Boffetta and Hashibe 2006), and for an association between BMI and lung cancer risk (WCRF 2007).

A positive familial history of lung cancer is a recognized risk factor. Segregation analyses suggest that inheritance of a major gene, in conjunction with tobacco smoking, might account for more than 50 % of cases diagnosed below age 60 (Gauderman et al. 1997). Genomewide association studies identified several high-risk variants, notably in genes involved in nicotine dependence and DNA repair (Truong et al. 2010).

There is conclusive evidence that exposure to ionizing radiation increases the risk of lung cancer (IARC 2000). Atomic bomb survivors and patients treated with radiotherapy for ankylosing spondylitis or breast cancer are at moderately increased risk of lung cancer, while studies of nuclear industry workers exposed to relatively low levels, however, provided no evidence of an increased risk of lung cancer. Underground miners exposed to radioactive radon and its decay products, which emit α-particles, have been found to be at increased risk of lung cancer (IARC 2001). The risk increased with estimated cumulative exposure and decreased with attained age and time since cessation of exposure (Lubin et al. 1994). Radon is an important cause of lung cancer also in circumstances of indoor air exposure, being responsible for an estimated 5–10 % of all lung cancers (Darby et al. 2005).

The risk of lung cancer is increased among workers employed in several industries and occupations. For several of these high-risk workplaces, the agent (or agents) responsible for the increased risk have been identified. Of these, asbestos, heavy metals and combustion fumes are the most important. Occupational agents are responsible for an estimated 5–10 % of lung cancers in industrialized countries.

Patients with pulmonary tuberculosis are at increased risk of lung cancer; it is not clear whether the excess risk is due to the chronic inflammatory status of the lung parenchima or to the specific action of the Mycobacterium. Chronic exposure to high levels of fibres and dusts might result in lung fibrosis (e.g., silicosis and asbestosis), a condition which entails an increase in the risk of lung cancer. Chronic bronchitis and emphysema have also been associated with lung cancer risk.

Lung cancer rates were higher in cities than in rural settings, particularly in the past (Hystad et al. 2013). Although this pattern might result from confounding by other factors, notably tobacco smoking and occupational exposures, the combined evidence from analytical studies suggests that urban air pollution might be a risk factor for lung cancer, although the excess risk is unlikely to be larger than 20 % in most urban areas.

Indoor air pollution is responsible for the elevated risk of lung cancer experienced by non-smoking women living in several regions of China and other Asian countries. The evidence is strongest for coal burning in poorly ventilated houses, but also burning of wood and other solid fuels, as well as fumes from high-temperature cooking using unrefined vegetable oils such as rapeseed oil (IARC 2010).

Control of tobacco smoking remains the key strategy for the prevention of lung cancer. Reduction in exposure to occupational and environmental carcinogens (in particular indoor pollution and radon), as well as increase in consumption of fruits and vegetables are additional preventive opportunities. Spiral CT scan has been shown to reduce lung cancer mortality (Aberle et al. 2011), although this effect needs to be assessed with respect to potential overdiagnosis of lung nodules with low malignant potential.

4.7.4 Pleural Mesothelioma

Mesothelioma is the most important primary tumour of the pleura. It can also originate from the peritoneum and the pericardium. Mesotheliomas were considered very rare tumours, until series of cases were reported in the 1960s among workers employed in to asbestos mining and manufacturing. The descriptive epidemiology of pleural tumours, and mesothelioma in particular, is complicated by geographical and temporal differences in diagnostic accuracy. In most high-resource countries, the incidence of pleural mesothelioma is in the order of 0.5–1/100,000 in men and around 0.2–0.4/100,000 in women. Lower rates are reported from low-resource countries, where under-diagnosis might be a particularly serious problem. In areas with a high prevalence of occupational exposure to asbestos such as shipbuilding and mining centres, the rates might be as high as 5/100,000 in men and 1/100,000 in women (Forman et al. 2013).

Occurrence of mesothelioma has been linked conclusively to expose to asbestos exposure, in particular to amphiboles such as crocidolite and amosite. Past occupational exposure to asbestos is the main determinant of pleural mesothelioma. High-exposure industries include mining, shipyard working, and mostly asbestos textile and cement manufacture (Boffetta and Stayner 2006).

Table 4.1 Observed and expected deaths form mesotelioma and lung cancer, and corresponding standardized mortality ratios (SMR) in relation to age at first and last employment[a]

	Person years	Mesothelioma			Lung cancer		
		Observed	Expected	SMR	Observed	Expected	SMR
First and last employment <30	30.366	25	0.4	6,626.7[b]	13	5.7	226.3[b]
First employment <30, last at age 30–39 years	6,035	9	0.11	8,019.0[b]	8	1.8	446.3[b]
First employment <30, last >40	2,832	6	0.10	5,896.0[b]	11	1.9	564.7[b]

[a]From Pira et al. (2007)
[b]Statistically significant ($p<0.05$)

Despite a reduction or ban of asbestos use in many countries, the incidence of mesothelioma has been increasing in the USA until the early 1990s, and in most Western European countries until the late 1990s, which reflects the long latency of the disease (Peto et al. 1999). The absolute risk (incidence) of mesothelioma in asbestos-exposed workers, in fact, is a function of dose, and of the third to fourth power of time since first exposure (Peto et al. 1982). Thus, time elapsed since first exposure (latency) is the major factor in defining subsequent mesothelioma risk, with an incidence over tenfold higher for a latency of 40 years compared with 25 years.

Data from five large studies published over the last decade (Table 4.1) (Pira et al. 2007; La Vecchia and Boffetta 2012) provide consistent evidence that for workers occupationally exposed in the distant past, the risk of mesothelioma is not appreciably influenced by subsequent exposures. Further, stopping exposure does not materially modify the risk of mesothelioma over subsequent decades. This is the reason for the still expanding mesothelioma epidemic across Europe (Peto et al. 1999), despite the appreciable decrease in exposure to asbestos since the 1970s, and the elimination of asbestos in most European countries since the early 1990s. In selected countries such as Sweden and US, however, rates have leveled off during the last decade (Hemminki and Hussain 2008; Moolgavkar et al. 2009).

In the absence of occupational exposure to asbestos, incidence rates on the order of 0.1–0.2/100,000 are estimated in both genders. There is evidence of an increased risk of pleural mesothelioma following environmental exposure to asbestos; epidemics of mesothelioma have been reported from areas with environmental contamination by other natural mineral fibers, such as some districts of central Turkey, where erionite, a fibrous substance similar to amphibole asbestos, contaminated the materials used for building construction.

In several populations, DNA of simian virus 40 has been reported in a high proportion of mesothelioma cases: however, a causal role of this virus, which contaminated polio vaccines used in the 1950s in many countries, has not been confirmed (Shah 2007). Exposure to ionizing radiation entails an increased risk of pleural mesothelioma, as it has been shown in cohorts of patients treated with thorotrast, a radiological contrast medium (Boffetta and Stayner 2006). Tobacco smoking, alcohol drinking and diet do not appear to be risk factors for pleural mesothelioma.

4.8 Neoplasms of the Bone and Soft Tissues

4.8.1 Bone Cancer

Three main histological types represent the majority of cases of bone cancer: osteosarcoma (originating from the bone tissue and representing 30–50 % of all bone neoplasms), chondrosarcoma (from the cartilage, 20–30 %) and Ewing's sarcoma (possibly from primitive nervous tissue, 10–20 %). Several other rare types (e.g., chordoma, fibrosarcoma, giant cell tumours) comprise some 10–20 % of all bone cancers. Ewing's sarcoma occurs mainly during the second and third decades of life; the incidence of osteosarcoma is bimodal with peaks between 10 and 30, and after age 60, while the incidence of chondrosarcoma resembles that of many cancers with a steady increase throughout life. Rates of all major histological types are higher in men than in women. In most populations the ratio is in the order of 1:1.5. There are limited geographical differences in bone cancer incidence, with rates ranging between 0.5 and 2/100,000 in men and between 0.5 and 1.5/100,000 in women (Forman et al. 2013).

Ionizing radiation is the best known risk factor for bone cancer (Miller et al. 2006). The risk is increased 2–3-fold in groups of adult patients undergoing radiotherapy for cancer, as compared to other patients: the RR is high among radiotherapy-treated children, in particular among those with inherited mutation in the RB gene, suggesting an interaction with genetic susceptibility. The excess risk, however, is apparent only among patients receiving high radiation doses (above 1,000 rad), and studies of populations exposed to lower doses, such as patients treated for benign conditions or atomic bomb survivors, did not show an increased risk. Studies of workers and patients exposed to high doses of radium isotopes also confirmed the role of ionizing radiation in bone carcinogenesis.

The evidence implying cancer chemotherapy, viral infections, traumas and medical implants is inadequate to reach a conclusion (Miller et al. 2006).

Patients with Paget's disease (osteitis deformans, a disease characterized by multiple localized areas of destruction of bone followed by repair) have a high incidence of osteosarcoma and chondrosarcoma: this disease is likely to be responsible for a substantial proportion of cases above age 60. A hereditary component of Paget's disease is suggested, and unknown environmental factors are likely to play a role in its aetiology. The risk of bone cancer is also increased in other rare syndromes of bone malformation. Bone cancer is one of the neoplasms appearing in the Li–Fraumeni syndrome, caused by an inherited mutation in the p53 gene, and other rare genetic syndromes. Familial aggregation of bone cancer occurs also outside well-defined inherited conditions, suggesting an important role of still unknown genetic factors.

The causes of Ewing's sarcoma are largely unknown. It is not associated with ionizing radiation and it does not appear to aggregate in families.

Primary prevention of bone cancer is hampered by the limited knowledge about its causes and mechanisms. No secondary prevention strategies are available.

4.8.2 Soft Tissue Sarcomas

Sarcomas originate from the mesenchyma in the space between the organs and within any organ. Sarcomas from the organs are classified within the neoplasms of that organ (e.g., liver angiosarcoma), while those originating from subcutaneous and intervisceral connective tissue are classified in the heterogeneous group of soft tissue sarcomas. Fibrosarcoma (originating from fibrocytes of the connective tissue), leiomyosarcoma (from smooth muscle cells) and liposarcoma (from fat cells) are common types of soft tissue sarcomas in most populations. The recent epidemic of AIDS has produced in several populations a sharp increase in the occurrence of Kaposi's sarcoma, a sarcoma from blood vessel cells (see below). Without considering Kaposi's sarcoma, the incidence of soft tissue sarcoma presents limited geographical variations, with age-adjusted incidence rates ranging from 1 to 4/100,000 in men and from 1 to 3/100,000 in women. Rates are slightly lower in Asia, and higher in Western Europe and North America (Forman et al. 2013). An increasing trend in incidence is suggested in high-resource countries, which is not explained by the increasing incidence of Kaposi's sarcoma, but might be caused by improved diagnosis and reporting.

Ionizing radiation is a known risk factor for soft tissue sarcomas: all types of sarcomas have been reported among patients treated with radiotherapy, the most frequent being malignant fibrous hystiocytoma (Berwick 2006). A viral agent (e.g., cytomegalovirus, EBV) has been hypothesized for non-AIDS related Kaposi's sarcoma and for other soft tissue sarcomas, but no conclusions can be reached at present.

There is no consistent evidence of an association with dietary factors, traumas, tobacco smoking or occupational exposures (Burningham et al. 2012).

Transplant patients receiving immunosuppressive therapy as well as patients with primary immunodeficiency syndromes have an increased risk of soft tissue sarcomas. The occurrence of these neoplasms is also increased in patients with the Li–Fraumeni syndrome, neurofibromatosis type 1 and other rare familial cancer syndromes. Benign tumours in the connective tissue (lipomas, fibromas, etc.) are common and usually do not transform into their malignant counterparts.

4.9 Cancer of the Skin

There are four main types of skin cancer: Squamous cell carcinoma (SqCC), arising from the epidermal cells, basal cell carcinoma (BCC), from basal cells forming sebaceous glands, melanoma, arising from melanocytes, and Kaposi's sarcoma, arising from endothelial cells. SqCC and BCC share some clinical and aetiological features, and are often combined under the definition of non-melanocytic skin cancer.

4.9.1 *Non-melanocytic Skin Cancer*

Given the simplified diagnostic and therapeutic procedures (often treated in outpatient clinics and physicians' offices) of most non-melanocytic skin cancers, and particularly of BCC, reporting of cases to registries is frequently incomplete, and many cancer registries do not attempt to provide incidence figures. The very good prognosis (a more than 95 % survival rate in most populations) makes mortality figures useless to estimate incidence particularly for BCC. Most population-based data incidence derive therefore from ad hoc surveys. One of these surveys conducted in the USA in the late 1970s estimated an age-adjusted incidence rate of SqCC of 68/100,000 in White men and 24/100,000 in White women; corresponding figures for BCC were 258 and 155/100,000. Rates in Blacks were about 100 times lower than in Whites, and SqCC predominates. The comparison with a similar survey conducted in the early 1970s revealed a 4–5 % increase in incidence of BCC per year, which can be attributed, at least in part, to improved diagnosis and surveillance procedures. SqCC rates increased little during the same period. The highest rates have been recorded in Ireland and among Whites living in countries with high solar exposure, such as Australia and South Africa, while Black populations have consistently low rates. Within Europe, the cancer registry from Vaud, Switzerland provided valid data on nonmelanomatoes skin cancer. BCC incidence tended to rise over research decades, to recent 77/100,000 men and 67 women, while that of SqCC levelled off around 29/100,000 for men and 17 for women (Levi et al. 2001). Subjects with a diagnosis of BCC had an exceedingly high rate of subsequent BCC, with a cumulative risk approaching 20 % at 20 years (Levi et al. 2006).

Between 75 and 90 % of both SqCC and BCC in Whites are localized on the face, head and neck. In Blacks, the lower extremities are the most frequent location of SqCC.

Solar radiation is the main risk factor for non-melanocytic skin cancer. For SqCC, the cumulative dose of ultraviolet (UV) radiation appears to be the predominant risk factor, while for BCC sun exposure and sunburning during childhood appear to be important determinants of subsequent risk. The effect of solar radiation has been shown following occupational, recreational and involuntary exposure. A strong excess of skin cancer has also been shown in psoriasis patients treated with psoralen in combination with UV radiation A. Solar keratosis is a precursor lesion of SqCC of the skin (not of basal cell carcinoma): it occurs in those areas of the skin exposed to solar radiation. The cumulative progression rate of keratosis to carcinoma (usually through a phase of carcinoma in situ, or Bowen's disease) is in the order of 5 %. Skin pigmentation is a modifying factor of the carcinogenic effect of UV radiation, with subjects with light pigmentation having the greatest risk (Karagas et al. 2006).

An excess risk of BCC, but not SqCC, has been shown following exposure to ionizing radiation (studies of medical personnel, uranium miners, radiotherapy patients and atomic bomb survivors): the shape of the dose–response appears to be linear without threshold (Levi et al. 2006). Exposure to arsenic and its inorganic compounds has been linked to an excess of skin cancer in people exposed occupationally, from drinking water or from drugs used in the past. Mixtures of polycyclic aromatic hydrocarbons (coal tar, tar pitch, soot, creosote, lubricating and cutting oils) are also carcinogenic to the skin: an excess of non-melanocytic cancer has been shown in classical occupational epidemiological studies among workers such as chimney sweeps, machine operators and roofers.

Skin cancer occurs in Asian countries as a consequence of burn scars produced by traditional heating devices kept in close contact to the skin: kangri in Kashmir, India, kairo in some areas of Japan and kang in northern China. It is possible that polycyclic aromatic hydrocarbons released by the burning material interact with heat in causing skin cancer. Tobacco smoking has not been associated to BCC, but is related to SqCC of the lip, and in—at least in the Nurses Health Study—to SqCC of other sites as well (Grodstein et al. 1995). Further, subjects diagnosed with SqCC have excess subsequent risk of tobacco-related cancers, as well as of lymphomas (Maitra et al. 2005).

Immunodeficiency increases the risk of SqCC of the skin, as it has been shown in patients treated with immunosuppressive drugs following renal transplant or other conditions. Xeroderma pigmentosum and the nevoid basal cell carcinoma syndrome are rare hereditary conditions characterized by a very high incidence of skin cancer. In the former syndrome, the mechanism is a reduced capacity to repair damage to DNA. The action of immunodeficiency and genetic predisposition may be via an enhancement of the carcinogenic effect of ultraviolet and ionizing radiation, since the neoplasms occur on parts of the body exposed to the sun.

4.9.2 Prevention of Non-melanocytic Skin Cancer

Avoidance of sun exposure, in particular during the middle of the day, is the primary preventive measure to reduce the incidence of skin cancer. There is no adequate evidence of a protective effect of sunscreens, possibly because use of sunscreens is associated with increased exposure to the sun. The possible benefit in reducing skin cancer risk by reduction of sun exposure, however, should be balanced against possible favourable effects of UV radiation in promoting vitamin D metabolism. Control of occupational skin carcinogens has taken place in many industries, although high exposure circumstances may still take place in a few low income countries. Control of exposure to sunshine in however still largely inadequate. Avoidance of drinking water with a high arsenic level should be a priority in contaminated areas for skin, but also for several other neoplasms, including lung and bladder (Steinmaus et al. 2013). Secondary prevention can be achieved by regular skin examination, in particular for high-risk individuals: however, there is a lack of controlled trials on skin cancer screening.

4.9.3 *Malignant Melanoma*

Malignant melanomas occur most frequently on the trunk in men and on the lower limbs in women. A special type of melanoma, is the rare lentigo malignant melanoma, which occurs on the head and neck, in areas with sun damage.

An estimated 230,000 new cases of malignant melanoma occurred worldwide in 2008 (Ferlay et al. 2013). The incidence is highest (in the order of 40/100,000) in men Western Australia, it ranges between 5 and 40/100,000 in other parts of Oceania, in North America and in Northern and Western Europe, and is below 5/1,000,000 in the other regions of the world. In general, the incidence is low in dark-skinned populations (Forman et al. 2013). In many White populations, there has been an increase in incidence and mortality of melanoma until the 1990s, with a recent levelling off: this pattern is inconsistent in non-White populations. Although part of this trend might be explained by increasing awareness and improved diagnosis, it is likely that it reflects to a large extent a true phenomenon. Studies of migrants have shown an increased risk following migration to a country with a sunny climate, such as Israel, South Africa and Australia. Age at migration is an important determinant of risk, since people who migrated at older age retain a risk similar to the risk of the country of origin, while younger migrants approach the risk of the host country. Melanoma shows a higher incidence in young adulthood than many other tumours. The increase with age is steeper for melanomas arising on the face, while the incidence of those on other parts of the body declines after middle age.

There is strong evidence of a carcinogenic role of ultraviolet radiation in determining malignant melanoma. Intermittent exposure to sun, and consequent sunburns, seems to play a more important role than total cumulative exposure.

Exposure to fluorescent lamp is not associated to the risk of melanoma, but artificial sources of Ultraviolet Radiation (UBV) have been related to excess risk.

Light colour of hair and eyes and skin complexion are risk factors for melanoma. Colour of hair seems to be the main predictor of risk, with RRs in the range of 1.5–2 for blond hair and 2–4 for red hair as compared to dark or brown hair. Freckling is likely to be an additional risk factor. Skin response to sun exposure and propensity to burn (or poor ability to tan) have also been associated to melanoma risk, with RRs in the range 1.5–4. However, pale complexion and propensity to burn are strongly correlated, and data are inadequate to completely separate these two factors.

Presence of a high number of nevi is the strongest risk factor for melanoma. Assessment of the number and type of nevi is not easy, and misclassification is likely to affect studies on nevi and melanoma. The RR is in the order of 10 for subjects with highest number of nevi. Their number depends on sun exposure, in particular intermittent exposure and sunburns: exposure in childhood is more important than exposure in adulthood. In subjects with familial melanoma, large atypical nevi, referred to as dysplastic nevi, may be found. Individuals with dysplastic nevi and familial melanoma have a very high risk of melanoma. In subjects without familial melanoma, presence of dysplastic nevi seems to be a risk factor independent from number of total nevi (Gruber and Armstrong 2006). The number of atypical nevi and the risk of melanoma are increased among immunosuppressed patients.

There is no clear evidence of a relevant role of any other risk factor, including diet and exogenous hormones, in the aetiology of melanoma. An inverse association has been registered for high consumption of carotenoids (Millen et al. 2004), but the findings are inconsistent (Naldi et al. 2004), and diet is therefore unlikely to be major determinants of skin melanoma on a population level. There is a 2–5-fold increased risk of melanoma in subjects with an affected relative, which is independent from exposure to solar radiation. Several putative high-risk genes have been proposed to explain the increased familial risk, in the absence however of definite findings.

Reducing of solar and other sources of UBV exposure, especially in childhood, is the major primary preventive measure. Early diagnosis, in particular of thin lesions, is associated with better survival: screening via medical examination is justified in high-risk individuals, defined according to familial history, type of skin and reaction to solar radiation.

4.9.4 Kaposi's Sarcoma

This form of slowly progressing cutaneous sarcoma of lymphoid origin was rare before the appearance of the Human Immunodeficiency Virus (HIV) epidemic, but was one of the major neoplasms assisted with HIV infection. The incidence of non-HIV-related Kaposi's sarcoma was highest in the Mediterranean basin and in Africa. The lesion is more frequent in rural than in urban areas.

Subjects (in particular homosexuals) infected with HIV have a high risk of Kaposi's sarcoma, i.e. about 10,000 times than non-HIV infected person. Kaposi's sarcoma herpes virus or human herpes virus 8, has been identified in HIV-positive cases (IARC 1996). The same virus has been detected in most analysed cases of non-HIV-related sarcoma and is likely to play a causal role in the development of most or all of Kaposi's sarcoma cases. The transmission of the herpes virus in HIV-infected individuals is likely to be via sexual contact: mode of transmission and cofactors in non-HIV individuals are not well understood.

4.10 Cancer of the Breast

Over 80 % of the neoplasms of the breast originate from the ductal epithelium, while a minority originates from the lobular epithelium. However, the proportion of ductal carcinomas has been increasing over recent calendar periods. Survival from breast cancer has slowly increased in high-resource countries, where it now achieves 85 %, following improvements in screening practices and treatments. Survival in low-resource countries remains poor, in the order of 50–60 %.

Breast cancer is the most common cancer among women worldwide: the estimated number of new cases in 2012 was 1,680,000 (800,000 in high-income and

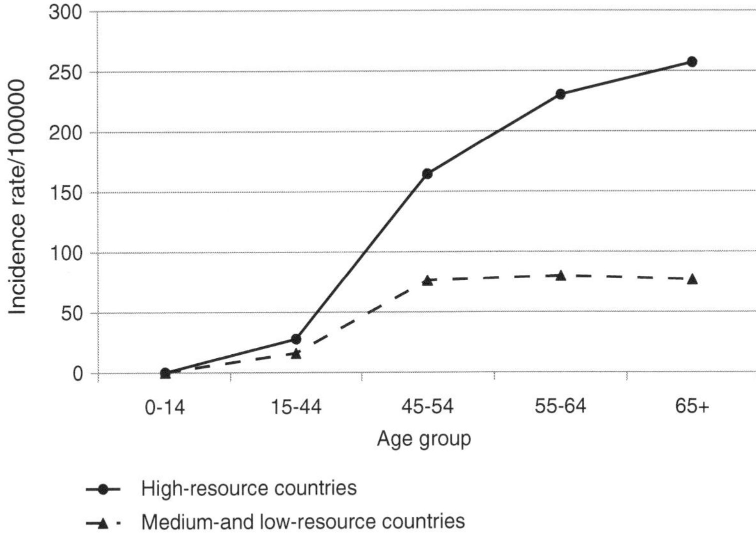

Fig. 4.4 Age specific incidence rates of breast cancer by region of the world, 2002 (Ferlay et al. 2010b)

980,000 low/middle-income countries) (Ferlay et al. 2013). It is also the most important cause of cancer deaths among women, causing an estimated 520,000 deaths. of which 3,200,000 in low- and middle-income countries. The incidence of breast cancer is low (less than 40/100,000) in most countries from sub-Saharan Africa, in China and in other countries of East Asia, except Japan, as well as the Caribbean and Northern countries of South America. The highest rates (90–100/100,000) are recorded in North America, Australia, and Northern and Western Europe (Forman et al. 2013) (Fig. 4.4). The incidence of breast cancer has grown rapidly during the last decades in many low-resource countries and slowly in middle- and high-resource countries. Mortality rates have remained fairly stable between 1960 and 1990 in most of Europe and the Americas, with however appreciable declines since the early 1990s, approaching 30 % in 2010 (Bosetti et al. 2013). The incidence increases linearly with age up to menopause, after which a further increase is less marked (high-resource countries) or almost absent (low-resource countries). Women from high social class have higher rates than women from low social class, the difference being in the order of 30–50 %.

In recent years there has been an increasing understanding of the etiologic heterogeneity of different subtypes of breast cancer, in addition to the importance of this classification for clinical and prognostic purposes. In addition to the distinction between pre- and post-menopausal cases, it has become clear the importance of hormone receptor status, with classification according to the presence of receptors for estrogen, progesterone and human epidermal growth factor 2 (Her2). Cases which are negative for the three receptors (so-called triple-negative breast cancers) are the least responsive to current therapies, and are those for which prevention would also be most effective in terms of impact of mortality. In addition, several types have been identified according to expression of various panels of genes: again, these classifications might guide future epidemiologic research on breast cancer.

The cumulative number of ovarian cycles is a determinant of breast cancer risk, and there is an increased risk for early age at menarche and late age at menopause. Artificial menopause exerts a similar or somewhat stronger protective effect than natural menopause (Colditz et al. 2006).

Pregnancy increases in the short term the risk of breast cancer, probably because of increase in the level of free estrogens during the first trimester. Overall, there is a protective role of early age at first pregnancy and a small residual protective effect of other pregnancies. An additional protective effect of lactation has been shown in several populations, which is probably attributable to the suppression of the ovulatory function caused by nursing. In a collaborative reanalysis of 47 studies, breast cancer risk decreased by 4 % for each year of lactation (Collaborative Group on Hormonal Factors Breast Cancer 2002). Epidemiological studies indicate a lack of association between spontaneous or induced abortions and breast cancer.

Current and recent users of OC have a modest increase (i.e., about 25 %) in risk of breast cancer as compared to never users. Further, 10 or more years after stopping use of OC the risk levels off to approach that of never users (IARC 2007b). This is of particular importance, since most women who use OC are young and have low baseline incidence of breast cancer. Therefore, their increased risk during and shortly after OC use is little relevant. With further reference to exogenous hormones, the evidence derived both from randomized clinical trials and observational epidemiological studies (cohort and case–control) indicates that the risk of breast cancer (mainly ductal cancer) is elevated among women using (combined) Hormonal Replacement Therapy (HRT) (IARC 2007b). Several epidemiological investigations consistently reported higher risks among current users of HRT, increasing from 1.1 to 1.6 according to their duration of use. The risk of breast cancer is reduced after cessation of use, and levels off after 5 or more years since quitting HRT. The Women's Health Initiative, a randomized controlled trial conducted on post-menopausal women, provided comprehensive information on the risk of breast cancer in users of conjugated estrogen alone or in combination with progestin. In the estrogen-alone trial, after about 7 years of follow-up, there was no significant difference in breast cancer incidence comparing conjugated estrogen users to the placebo group (Stefanick et al. 2006). On the other hand, a higher incidence of invasive breast cancer was observed in the estrogen plus progestin group as compared to women receiving placebo. Further, breast cancers were diagnosed at a more advanced stage in the estrogen plus progestin group (Chlebowski et al. 2003).

The combined evidence from reproductive factors points towards an important role of endogenous hormones in breast carcinogenesis. A direct assessment of the role of estrogen and testosterone is also available from recent prospective studies collecting data of biological samples. Estradiol concentrations in the blood have been directly associated with breast cancer risk in post-menopausal women, whereas data are fewer and results are less consistent in pre-menopausal women. The association might be stronger with estrogen and progesterone receptor positive tumors. Comparable findings have been reported for measures of testosterone and other androgens, but the data are inconsistent for all endogenous hormones across major cohort studies.

Women suffering from the two most common benign breast diseases, fibrocystic disease and fibroadenoma carry a 2–3-fold increased risk of breast cancer. While these lesions are not likely to represent pre-neoplastic conditions, they share with breast cancer epithelial proliferation, linked to hormonal alterations. A related risk factor is breast density, a measure used to describe the proportion of breast and connective tissue seen on a mammogram compared to fat. Despite the inherent imprecision of the measurement of breast density, this characteristics has been consistently reported to predict breast cancer risk, with an estimated 16 % of breast cancer attributable to high mammographic density (Assi et al. 2012).

A history of breast cancer in first degree relatives is associated with a 2–3-fold increased risk of the disease. Most of the role of familial history is likely to result from low-penetrance genes associated with hormonal metabolism and regulation, DNA damage and repair. A number of genomewide association studies have identified over 50 variants which appear to modify the susceptibility to breast cancer, each conferring a modest excess risk (in the order of 10–25 %): some of the genes are involved in DNA repair and cell cycle control, but the functional role of most variants remains unclear (Peng et al. 2011). Specific sets of variants have been identified for subpopulations, such as Asian women, and cases of triple negative breast cancer. In addition, breast cancer risk is greatly increased in carriers of mutations of several high-penetrance genes, in particular *BRCA1*, *BRCA2*, *ATM*, *CHECK2* and *p53*. Although the cumulative lifetime risk in carriers of these genes is over 50 %, they are rare in most populations and explain only a small fraction (2–5 %) of total cases. There are exceptions, however, such as Ashkenazi Jews, among whom high-risk *BRCA1* or *BRCA2* mutations are responsible for an estimated 12 % of breast cancers.

Although a role of nutrition in breast cancer risk is strongly suggested by international comparisons, the combined evidence from epidemiological studies is inconclusive for most aspects of diet, including intake of fruit and vegetables, total fat, saturated fat and fibres (WCRF 2007). Similarly, results on micronutrients have been elusive, although there is some evidence of a protective role played by folate and phytoestrogens, particularly isoflavones and dietary lignans. Further, vitamin D, and in particular serum 25(OH) D levels, have been inversely related to breast cancer risk (Giovannucci 2005). Hormonal levels and nutritional factors during the intrauterine period and childhood are also likely to be important in breast carcinogenesis. In fact, energy intake during childhood is one of the determinant of adult height, which in turn has been directly associated with breast cancer risk in most epidemiological studies.

Besides height, other anthropometric factors are involved in the aetiology of breast cancer. Reduced energy intake in early life is associated with a smaller body size, which likely entails a reduced breast cancer risk (Lagiou et al. 2006). An increased risk with increasing weight during adult life has been consistently reported among women older than 60, but not among younger women. Body mass index is associated to breast cancer, the relation being inverse in pre-menopausal and direct in post-menopausal women (WCRF 2007). Several studies reported a modifying effect of HRT use on the relation between body weight and weight gain and breast cancer in post-menopausal women. The increase in risk of breast cancer observed for a high body weight and/or weight gain was stronger or limited to non-users of HRT (La Vecchia 2007).

Many lifestyle factors have been investigated as possible causes of breast cancer. Alcohol drinking is an established aetiological factor. Consumption of three or more alcoholic drinks per day carries an increased risk in the order of 30–50 %, with each daily drink accounting for an about 7 % higher risk. It is likely that both overweight and heavy alcohol drinking act on breast cancer through mechanisms involving hormonal level or metabolism. Tobacco smoking or second-hand tobacco smoke do not appear to carry an increased risk of breast cancer. A high level of physical activity, on the other hand, is likely to moderately decrease the risk. Studies of occupational factors and of exposure to organic chemicals have failed to provide evidence of an aetiological role.

Less than 1 % of all cases of breast cancer occur in men. The incidence provides limited evidence of geographical and interracial variations, with no clear correlation with incidence in women. Conditions involving high oestrogen level, such as gonadal dysfunction, alcohol abuse and obesity, are risk factors for breast cancer in men. BRCA2 mutations are more frequent than BRCA1 in male familial breast cancers.

4.10.1 Prevention of Breast Cancer

Primary prevention of breast cancer has been attempted via nutritional intervention, involving reduction of energy intake, reduction of proportion of calories from fat, and increase in fruit and vegetable consumption. No evidence of efficacy has been produced so far. However, control of weight gain and of overweight and obesity or postmenopausal women would have favourable implications in breast cancer risk.

Tamoxifen, an anti-oestrogen drug used in chemotherapy, has shown a chemopreventive action against breast cancer, although its use is recommended in women with a previous breast cancer only. Aspirin and other nonsteroidal anti-inflammatory drugs might also have a chemopreventive effect on breast cancer risk, although results from epidemiological studies are heterogeneous (Bosetti et al. 2012d).

The most suitable approach for breast cancer control is secondary prevention through mammography. Breast cancer screening began to be implemented in the late 1980s. The effectiveness of screening by mammography in women older than 50 years has been demonstrated, and programmes have been established in various countries, although some controversies remain in the interpretation of the available evidence (IUKPBCS 2012). The reduction in mortality, typically of the order of

25 % seen in RCTs, are not replicated in routine screening where the reductions are more often in the range of 5–15 % in the general population 15–20 years after full rollout of the programme (Anttila et al. 2008; Kalager et al. 2010). The effectiveness in women younger than 50 is not yet demonstrated, though there is some evidence for a reduction in risk of dying from breast cancer in women aged 40–49 years that undergo annual mammography.

Other screening techniques, including breast self examination, have not been proven to reduce breast cancer mortality.

4.11 Cancer of the Female Genital Organs

The female genital organs comprise the ovaries and their annexes, the uterus, the vagina and the external genitals. The uterus is composed of two parts, the cervix and the corpus, which have distinct physiological and pathological features. Cancers of the cervix and corpus of the uterus are different histologically, clinically and aetiologically. However, the distinction between cervix and corpus is often neglected in records used for epidemiological purposes, and particular in death certificates from several countries. Today in Europe and North America, most cancers of the uterus without further specification are likely to be cancer of the corpus. This, however, may not have been the case in the past, and particularly in middle and low income countries, and this complicates the interpretation of temporal trends and geographical comparisons.

4.11.1 Cancer of the Uterine Cervix

Cervical cancer is a major public health problem in many low and middle income countries. Incidence rates are high (20–40/100,000) in sub-Saharan Africa and Latin America countries, as well as in India and southern Asia. In China, the Middle East, northern Africa and high-income countries, rates are in the order of 5–15/100,000 (Forman et al. 2013). This results in a number of cases each year in excess of 520,000. Of these, more than 85 % of which occur in low and middle income countries. The number of estimated cancer deaths in low- and middle-income countries (230,000 in 2012) is second to breast cancer only (320,000) (Ferlay et al. 2013). Incidence and mortality rates have decreased steadily in high-income countries, but an upturn in incidence had been observed among young women in a few of these. Few data on temporal trends are available from middle and low income countries, but incidence has likely decreased during recent decades in those areas of the world, too. In high income countries, rates increase up to age 60, while in middle and low income countries there is little increase above age 50. Cervical cancer hits preferentially women of lower education and social class.

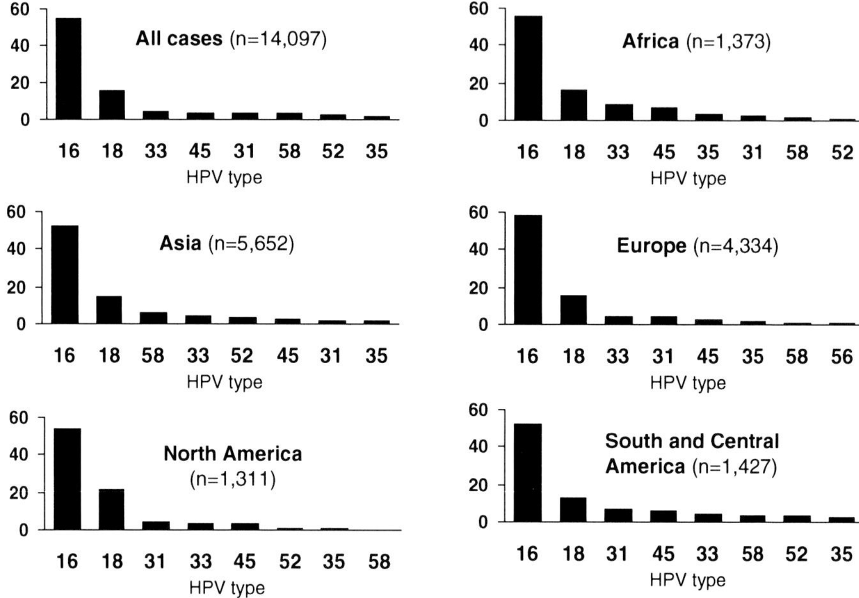

Fig. 4.5 Most common HPV types in 14,097 cases of invasive cervical cancer by region (Smith et al. 2007)

Most cervical cancers originate from the area of squamous metaplasia called transformation zone, which is adjacent to the junction between the columnar epithelium of endometrial origin and the cheratinizing epithelium of vaginal origin. Most invasive cancers are SqCC or mixed adeno-squamous tumours. Invasive carcinoma is preceded by inflammatory and condylomatous atypia, mild dysplasia (also called cervical intraepithelial neoplasia of grade 1, or CIN 1), moderate dysplasia (CIN 2), severe dysplasia and carcinoma in situ (CIN 3) (Schiffman and Hildesheim 2006).

Chronic infection with HPV is a necessary cause of cervical cancer. Using sensitive molecular techniques, virtually all tumours are positive for the virus, (Clifford et al. 2005; Smith et al. 2007). Different types of HPV exist, and those associated with cervical cancer are mainly types 16, 18, 31, 45 and 58. In particular, HPV 16 is the main cervical carcinogen in most populations, while the distribution of other types varies by geographical region (Fig. 4.5). Differences in prevalence of HPV infection explain much of the descriptive epidemiology of cervical cancer (geographical patterns, high risk in low social class, etc.). The host response to HPV infection is important in determining its carcinogenic effect; immunosuppression, as present in transplanted patients and HIV infected individuals, increases the risk of dysplasia, carcinoma in situ, and invasive neoplasms.

Sexual histories of women (early age at first intercourse and high number of sexual partners) and of their male partners (high number of sexual partners, presence of genital diseases and contact with prostitutes) are risk factors for cervical cancer in many populations. They reflect an increased likelihood of HPV infection, as well as the duration of HPV infection. As for most carcinogens, in fact, duration of exposure is the major determinant of subsequent cancer risk (La Vecchia et al. 1986; Peto 2012; Plummer et al. 2012).

Studies of infection with other agents, in particular Chlamydia and Herpes Simplex 2, have failed to provide consistent evidence of an effect independent from HPV. An increased risk, of the order of twofold, has been detected among long-term current or recent users of OC, which is not completely explained by sexual behaviour or HPV infection. However, there is no residual association 5–10 years after stopping OC use. Consequently, the public health implications of OC use on cervical cancer risk are limited in time (La Vecchia and Bosetti 2003; Bosetti et al. 2005; Appleby et al. 2007; Cibula et al. 2010). Condom and (perhaps) diaphragm, on the other hand, exert a protective effect, possibly via prevention of HPV infection.

Tobacco smoking has also an independent effect on cervical carcinogenesis with a RR of 1.5–1.6 for current smokers, also once HPV infection is taken into account (IARC 2004). A possible protective effect of a diet rich in fruits and vegetables has been suggested in a few studies, but the role of diet on cervical cancer risk is probably modest and largely undefined.

Cytological examination of exfoliated cervical cells (the Papanicolaou smear, PAP test) is effective in identifying precursor lesions, resulting in a substantial decrease in incidence of and mortality from invasive cancer. Cytological smears are not largely applicable, however, in countries with limited availability of cytologists and pathologists, including in many countries with high prevalence of HPV infection and high incidence of invasive cancer. Alternative approaches for secondary prevention have therefore been proposed, including visual inspection of the cervix with possible enhancement of precursor lesions by acetic acid, but their efficacy on cervical cancer prevention remains unproven. Use of HPV testing appears now however to be more specific and sensible than that the PAS test, and is therefore likely to replica PAS smear as the first screening method in the near future. The primary method for prevention of cervical cancer for future generations, however, is likely to become HPV vaccination. One vaccine against HPV 16, 18 (as well, 6 and 11, linked to genital warts) is now available, and another against HPV 16 and 18 only (FUTURE II Study Group 2007). Vaccine including larger numbers of HPV strains (i.e., 8 strains) are in the late stage of testing. The final impact of the effect of such vaccination is complicated by the geographical variations in the distribution of HPV types (Cuzick 2010).

4.11.2 Cancer of the Uterine Corpus

Cancer of the endometrium is the most frequent malignant neoplasm of the uterine corpus, while sarcomas, originating from the connective muscular tissue, are relatively rare. The descriptive epidemiology of cancer of the uterine corpus is complicated by the large proportion of hysterectomized women in high-income countries.

The number of new cases occurring in 2008 worldwide was estimated in the order of 170,000, of which two-thirds occurred in high-income countries (Ferlay et al. 2010a). The number of deaths is in the order of 70,000. Incidence rates are relatively high (10–20/100,000) in Europe and North America, while they are below 5/100,000 in most African countries (Forman et al. 2013), in the Caribbean, and in most areas of China. Endometrial cancer is a neoplasm of postmenopausal women. In the USA, the incidence (but not mortality) is higher in Whites as compared to Blacks (IARC 2007a).

Nulliparity, infertility and late age at menopause are associated with a 2–3-fold increased risk of endometrial cancer. The evidence regarding other reproductive factors, including early age at menarche, is less consistent. Medical conditions resulting in high endogenous oestrogen levels (including oestrogen-secreting tumours and polycystic ovarian syndrome, particularly in obese women) have been consistently associated to an increased endometrial cancer risk. Studies of blood oestrogen levels, however, are too sparse to be conclusive (Cook et al. 2006).

An increased risk of endometrial cancer was reported in the 1970s in the USA, followed by a decline up to the 1990s. This trend in incidence parallels the patterns of postmenopausal unopposed oestrogen use. Use of oestrogen replacement therapy is associated with a twofold increase in risk of endometrial cancer. The strength of the association depends on the dose and the duration of use. Addition of progestin to oestrogen replacement therapy protects from the increased risk of endometrial cancer, but it increases the risk of breast cancer and cardiovascular disease (Chlebowski et al. 2003; IARC 2007b). An increased risk of endometrial cancer has also been shown among breast cancer patients treated with tamoxifen at a relatively high dosage (30–40 mg) or for a long period of time (5 or more years), though results are not consistent for low dosages and short period of tamoxifen use. Combined contraceptives, on the other hands, reduce the risk of endometrial cancer by about 50 % and the protection is long lasting (Cibula et al. 2010).

An increased risk of endometrial cancer has been consistently reported among obese women as compared to lean ones (IARC 2002). Depending on the measure used to evaluate overweight, endometrial cancer risk increases 2–10-fold. An increased risk in the order of 50–100 % has also been reported among women with diabetes and perhaps hypertension, which does not seem to be fully explained by increased weight in these patients. A decreased risk of endometrial cancer has been reported among smokers, particularly among post-menopausal women: this result has been attributed to an anti-oestrogenic or pro-androgenic activity of smoking. The results of studies of diet and endometrial cancer have been inconsistent. Several other potential risk factors have been addressed, including alcohol and coffee drinking, selected aspects of diet—besides overweight and obesity, and history of gallbladder disease, without however conclusive evidence of an association.

Current knowledge suggests that an impact on primary prevention of endometrial cancer can be made by avoidance of overweight and by minimizing the use of unopposed oestrogens.

4.11.3 Ovarian Cancer

Most malignant neoplasms of the ovary originate from the coelomic epithelium; less frequent tumours originate from the germ cells (dysgerminomas and teratomas) and the follicular cells (granulosa cell tumours). The estimated number of new cases worldwide in 2008 was in the order of 240,000, that of deaths of 150,000 (Ferlay et al. 2013). High incidence rates (in the order of 7–11/100,000) are found in Western and Northern Europe, in North America and Argentina; the lowest rates (below 3/100,000) are from China and most Africa (Forman et al. 2013). In high-risk countries, incidence rates have remained stable in recent decades, but mortality has tended to decline.

Early age at menarche is a risk factor, but its effect on ovarian cancer risk is modest. Lifelong number of menstrual cycles has also been associated with ovarian cancer risk, suggesting that ovulation is implicated in the process of ovarian carcinogenesis, but the contribution of parity and OC appears to be greater than that of other factors (Pelucchi et al. 2007). Several studies showed a direct relation between late age at menopause and the risk of ovarian cancer (Hankinson and Danforth 2006).

Nulliparity and low parity are related to ovarian cancer. Most studies showed a decline in risk associated with number of full-term pregnancies beyond the first one, thus suggesting that additional risk reduction is conferred by each pregnancy.

The protection afforded by combined OC is also established, and is most important from a public health perspective, feature of epithelial ovarian cancer. The overall estimated protection is approximately 40 % in ever OC users and increases with duration of use. The favorable effect of OC against ovarian cancer risk persists for at least 30 years after OC use has ceased, and it is not confined to any particular type of OC formulation (La Vecchia et al. 2001; Collaborative Group on Epidemiological Studies of Ovarian Cancer et al. 2008; Cibula et al. 2010) . Women who had used OC for 15 years have a 0.5 % reduced cumulative incidence of ovarian cancer to age 75, and a 0.3 % reduced mortality. The issue of fertility drugs and ovarian cancer has also attracted interest, but the findings remain inconsistent. Use of HRT in menopause has been related to increased ovarian cancer risk, by about 50 % for 5 years of use (La Vecchia 2006; IARC 2007b).

Potential links between ovarian cancer and diet were originally suggested on the basis of international differences and correlation studies. A relation between ovarian cancer and intake of meat and fats has also been reported from some cohort and case–control studies, whereas fruit and vegetables appear to be inversely related. Some case–control studies found direct associations between measures of fat intake and risk of ovarian cancer. Starchy foods, and consequently diets with a high glycemic index and glycemic load, have also been related to excess ovarian cancer risk. The possibility that milk sugar lactose, or its metabolites, have some effect on oocytes with a compensatory gonadotropic stimulation and excess ovarian cancer risk has been investigated. Several, but not all, studies have found excess risk with lactose consumption and absorption, but the issue remains unsettled. Studies from

Greece and Italy suggested that monounsaturated fats (olive oil) and fiber intake may be favorable. The role of diet on ovarian cancer incidence and mortality rates and trends remains, however, unquantified. However, height and overweight were associated with excess ovarian cancer risk. Data for a pooled analysis including 25,157 cases give a RRs of 1.07 for 5 cm of height and of 1.10 for 5 kg/m^2 increase in BMI in never users of HRT only (Collaborative Group on Epidemiological Studies of Ovarian Cancer 2012).

Tobacco smoking is associated with mucinous, but not with other histological types of ovarian cancer (Collaborative Group on Epidemiological Studies of Ovarian Cancer et al. 2012).

There have long been clinical observations suggesting familial aggregations of ovarian cancer. Besides the clustering of ovarian cancer, an excess of breast cancer and a more general excess of several cancers (including colon and endometrium) have been described. These patterns are consistent with an autosomal dominant gene with variable penetration. The estimated RR from case–control studies that included data on family history range between 3 and 5. Two tumour-suppressor genes have been identified, BRCA1 on chromosome 17q and BRCA2 on chromosome 13q, whose autosomal dominant transmitted mutations confer a high risk of breast and ovarian cancer. BRCA1 may account for 5 % of ovarian cancers below age 50, and 2 % between age 50 and 70 (Negri et al. 2003).

The prevention of ovarian cancer—apart from the chemopreventive effect of OC use—which however is not applicable on a population level—is currently hampered by the limited knowledge of its causes and the lack of availability of early diagnostic techniques.

4.11.4 Cancer of Vagina and Vulva

The incidence of vaginal and vulvar cancers ranges between 0.5 and 4.5/100,000: high rates are reported from Europe and North America, while low rates are recorded in Eastern Asia (Forman et al. 2013). The incidence of vulvar cancer is about three times that of vaginal cancer. They are mainly SqCC; rare types are melanoma, sarcoma and clear cell adenocarcinoma.

Infection with HPV is the best recognised risk factor for these cancers, with a RR of 10 or greater (Madeleine and Daling 2006). HPV 16 is the most commonly reported type. Other sexually transmitted diseases, including syphilis, Herpes Simplex type 2, and lymphogranuloma venereum have been suggested as risk factors, but a confounding effect of HPV infection cannot be excluded.

Pelvic irradiation for cervical cancer or other diseases is another risk factor for vaginal and vulvar cancers. The occurrence of these neoplasms is associated with the presence of other cancers in the anogenital tract; this phenomenon might be explained by HPV infection at several sites. An association between tobacco smoking and vulvar and vaginal cancers has also been suggested.

Control of HPV infection is likely to be the key primary preventive measure for these, as well as other anogenital cancers.

Clear cell adenocarcinoma of the vagina is a rare tumour occurring in girls and young women, mainly following in utero exposure to diethylstilbestrol, a synthetic oestrogen used between the 1940s and the mid 1950s in North America and in several countries of western Europe. An increased risk in the order of twofold has also been reported for SqCC of the vagina and cervix.

4.11.5 Choriocarcinoma

Choriocarcinoma is a rare cancer that originates from the trophoblastic epithelium of the placenta. It is very aggressive, but most cases respond to chemotherapy. In most populations the incidence rate is in the range 0.1–0.5/100,000, although comparisons are complicated by diagnostic and reporting procedures (Forman et al. 2013).

Late material age is associated to gestational throphoblastic diseases, and the strongest risk factor for choriocarcinoma is hydatidiform mole, a benign gestational trophoblastic disease, which, in its complete form, occurs in the preceding pregnancy of 40–50 % of cases of choriocarcinoma (Altieri et al. 2003; Palmer and Feltmate 2006). The role of other reproductive factors, including infertility, number of pregnancies, and age at pregnancy, is unclear. There is evidence, albeit based on a relatively small number of studies, that use of OC is associated to both mole and carcinoma.

4.12 Cancer of the Male Genital Organs

4.12.1 Prostate Cancer

Cancer of the prostate is the most common malignant neoplasm in men from North America, where the incidence is as high as 130/100,000 and Brazil where it reaches 150/100,000. In Europe the incidence varies widely, from 30–140/100,000, while in most low- and middle-income countries it is below 30/100,000, and it can be as low as 10/100,000 in Southern and Eastern Asia (Forman et al. 2013). The estimated number of new cases occurring worldwide in 2012 was over 1,100,000 (Ferlay et al. 2013). Mortality rates show less variability among regions, suggesting that the number of non-fatal cases diagnosed in different countries varies depending on screening and other diagnostic procedures. The estimated number of deaths is over 300,000, less than 50 % of which occur in high-income countries. The incidence of prostate cancer increased during the last decades in most populations; in the USA and Canada, and subsequently in Europe and other high-income regions of the world, a very rapid increase has been observed since the mid 1980s. The disease is more common in African Americans than in while Americans. In most countries, it is more common among affluent groups of the population.

The descriptive epidemiology (incidence) of prostate cancer is highly dependent on the adoption of Prostate Specific Antigen (PSA) testing. Prostate cancer incidence has shown substantial changes following the introduction of PSA testing, with major increases due to the detection of large number of prevalent cases, followed by substantial declines. The changes in trends have been much smaller for mortality, but both in the USA and in Western Europe, peak rates were observed in the early 1990s, with a leveling off and a decline thereafter, approaching 20 % in the EU (La Vecchia et al. 2010; Bosetti et al. 2011; Bosetti et al. 2013).

The recent trends in prostate cancer mortality in Europe are consistent with a favorable impact of improved diagnosis, and well as of advancements in therapy, on prostate cancer mortality in Western Europe and North America.

Prospective studies failed to provide convincing evidence of an increased risk linked to increased level of testosterone or other sexual hormones. Similarly, an increased risk of prostate cancer was reported in retrospective studies following history of benign prostatic hypertrophy, but no excess risk was found in prospective studies. If an association exists between prostatic hypertrophy and cancer, it can be due to shared aetiological factors or to a common pathological process.

Carriers of *BRCA1* and *BRCA2* mutations have a 4–5-fold increased risk of prostate cancer. More in general, history of prostate cancer in first-degree relatives carries a 2–3-fold increased risk of developing the same neoplasm. Similar associations, of smaller magnitude, are also suggested for family history of breast and colon cancers (Negri et al. 2005). Genetic variants entailing an increased risk of prostate cancer have been identified within the 8q24 region (Amundadottir et al. 2006; Gudmundsson et al. 2007a, b; Haiman et al. 2007; Yeager et al. 2007) and possibly the 17q12 region (Gudmundsson et al. 2007b).

It has been suggested that the risk of the disease increases with number of sexual partners and number of encounters with prostitutes, and with previous history of syphilis and gonorrhoea. Serological studies of HPV 16 and HPV 18 have shown an increased risk among positive subjects, but the findings are inconsistent. It is not clear at present, however, whether syphilis and HPV are causal factors or markers of infection with sexually transmitted agents, and hence general markers of inflammation.

A possible protective role of high intake of vegetables has been suggested in a few studies; high intake of meat, diary products, total fat and saturated fat might represent a risk factor. The evidence concerning other dietary factors, including fruit intake and intake of specific micronutrients, is however largely inconclusive at present. These include lycopene, a retinoid present in particular in tomatoes which has been found to be associated with a reduced risk in a few (but not other) studies, and calcium which has been associated with elevated risk, possibly on account of its influence on vitamin D balance. There is in fact biological evidence that the most active form of vitamin D, 25 (OH) D, has a favourable role on prostate cancer, but epidemiological data are inconsistent (Giovannucci 2005). Vitamin D may prevent prostate cancer progression, and hence the most aggressive forms of the disease (Li et al. 2007), and there is also a suggestion of an increased risk among individuals with elevated serum level of insulin-like growth factor 1. An increased risk of the disease has been repeatedly reported among subjects with a high weight or body mass (Platz and Giovannucci 2006). Data on nutrition, diet and prostate cancer, are however largely inconsistent.

4.12.2 *Prevention of Prostate Cancer*

Still, the wide geographical variability of prostate cancer suggests that environmental factors likely related to diet and other lifestyle factors, such as physical activity, are important determinants of the disease. Primary prevention, however, is hampered by the fragmentary knowledge of its precise causes. Secondary prevention has been proposed, based on measurement of PSA and digital rectal examination. There is little evidence from controlled trials that either procedure decreases the mortality from prostate cancer (Boyle and Brawley 2009; Welch and Albertsen 2009). Despite this lack of evidence, these procedures, in particular the PSA testing, have gained popularity in many countries, and are the cause of the steep increase in number of diagnosed cased since the mid 1980s in North America and other high-income countries. It is unclear how much of the decrease in mortality reported since the mid 1990s in the USA and in Western Europe can be attributed to a beneficial effect of (unplanned) use of PSA testing, but it is likely due mainly to improved management and treatment of the disease, including better surgery, radiotherapy and medical therapy.

4.12.3 *Testicular Cancer*

Some 95 % of malignant neoplasms of the testis arise from the germinal tissue. About half of the germinal neoplasms are seminomas, while the remaining comprise teratomas and a variety of rare lesions. Testicular cancer is common in young age, and its incidence decreases after age 30. Teratomas and other non-seminomatous neoplasms predominate before age 15, after which most tumours are seminomas. Incidence rates are high (up to 10/100,000) in Latin America and Western Europe (up to 10/100,000) and are low (1/100,000 or less) in most of Africa and in Eastern and Southern Asia. In the USA, rates are higher in European Americans than in African Americans (Forman et al. 2013). The global number of incident cases in 2012 has been estimated at 55,000, that of deaths at 10,000 (Ferlay et al. 2013). The incidence has increased in most countries during the last decades, with evidence of a birth cohort effect. In many countries, the risk if higher in the more affluent groups of the population.

Cryptorchism is the best recognised cause of testicular cancer (Sarma et al. 2006). The RR is in the order of 2–5; this risk factor might be responsible for up to 10 % of all cases of testicular cancer. The risk is lower when orchiopexy is performed before age 10 than at older ages (Pettersson et al. 2007). This suggests that temperature and other micro-environmental factors might be responsible for the development of cancer in the undescended testis. Several rare diseases affecting gonadal differentiation, including Klinefelter's syndrome, increase the risk of non-germinal tumours of the testis. Exposure to elevated oestrogen levels during pregnancy, from either endogenous or exogenous origin, might be a risk factor for testicular cancer, although the evidence of an association is not consistent among studies. Familial aggregation has also been shown for different types of testicular cancer.

The limited knowledge about the causes of testicular cancer makes it difficult to devise effective preventive strategies, with the exception of early surgical treatment of cryptorchism.

Testicular cancer, particularly seminomas and teratomas in young men, is one of the most curable neoplasms, if adequate treatment is adopted. Substantial differences in mortality from this neoplasm were found between Western and Eastern European countries, probably due to different availability of the (expensive) drugs required to treat testicular cancer, as well as the attitudes and general capacity of various health systems to menage testicular cancer using up to date integrated therapeutic approaches (Levi et al. 2003; La Vecchia et al. 2010; Bosetti et al. 2011; Bosetti et al. 2013). Likewise, mortality from testicular cancer substantially declined in North America, but less so in Central and South America, though notes are now leveling up in the young (Bertuccio et al. 2007). Widespread adoption of efficacious therapy worldwide is therefore a priority to avoid unnecessary deaths from testicular cancer in young men.

4.12.4 Cancer of the Penis

Cancer of the penis comprises mainly SqCC, which is commonly preceded by intraepithelial lesions, including Queyrat's erythroplasia and Bowen's disease. The neoplasm in more common (rates in the order of 2–4/100,000) in Latin America and in South and South-East Asia, and is rare (0.5–1/100,000) in North America and Europe (Forman et al. 2013). In high-resource countries, incidence declined during the last decades (Ferlay et al. 2010a).

Chronic infection with HPV is the most important risk factor for penile cancer: the proportion of positive cases is in the order of 90 % (Widerof and Schottenfeld 2006). HPV type 16 is the most frequently found, followed by types 18, 45, and 31. Although the distribution of penile cancer and penile intraepithelial neoplasia parallels the distribution of the corresponding cervical lesions in women, their incidence is generally lower, suggesting differences either in tissue susceptibility or in the role played by cofactors.

A decreased risk of penile cancer has been reported among circumcized men, in particular among those operated in infancy. The most likely explanation of this effect is a protection against HPV infection. Furthermore, a high risk of penile cancer has been found among men with phimosis, in particular when it is associated with balanoposthisis (inflammation of the glans and prepuce).

Patients treated with oral 8-methoxypsoralen and ultraviolet A radiation (PUVA) for psoriasis or other skin disorders are at increased risk of penile and scrotal cancer. The carcinogenic effect is attributable to the combination therapy rather than to the skin disease.

Prevention of HPV infection through vaccination would be an effective preventive measure for penile cancer, though no direct data on the issue are available. Vaccination of girl is likely to substantially reduce penile cancer incidence in future cohorts of eterosexual men. HPV testing might be used for screening of high-risk individuals. A beneficial preventive effect of circumcision is probable, but remains unquantified.

4.13 Cancer of the Urinary Organs

The urinary organs comprise the kidneys (renal parenchyma), renal pelvis, ureter, urinary bladder and urethra. The majority of urinary cancers occur in the renal parenchyma and the bladder. Cancers of the renal pelvis, ureter and urethra are much rarer and less well studied and are, for statistical purposes, often grouped under kidney cancers. However, these tumours are histologically more similar to those of the bladder than the renal parenchyma, and their aetiology is also likely to be similar to that of bladder cancer.

4.13.1 Cancer of the Urinary Bladder

Bladder cancer accounts for approximately two-thirds of all urinary tract cancers with 430,000 cases worldwide in 2012, 60 % of which occurred in high-resource countries (Ferlay et al. 2013). The male-to-female ratio of 2–3 to 1 is higher than for kidney cancer. The vast majority of bladder cancers are transitional cell carcinomas, with the exception of bladder cancers related with schistosomiasis infection, which are mainly SqCC. High bladder cancer rates (30/100,000 or more in men) are observed in Southern and Western Europe, and intermediate rates (20–30/100,000 in men) in other parts of Europe, USA and Australia, as well as in Israel, Egypt and Uruguay. These high rates generally reflect those countries with high levels of cigarette smoking in the past, with the exception of Egypt where the high incidence is due to infection with Schistosoma. Bladder cancer incidence is complicates to evaluate, since the distinction between bladder papillomas and carcinomas is difficult in cancer registration. Mortality, however, is a more valid indicator, and has been declining in North America, Western Europe and Japan over the last two decades (Pelucchi et al. 2006).

Tobacco smoking is the single best recognized risk factor for bladder cancer, with RR up to fourfold elevated in heavy smokers (Gandini et al. 2008), and estimated attributable risk proportions in the order of 55 % in men and 20 % in women.

Thus, the decline in smoking prevalence in men from most Western—and, subsequently, Central and Eastern European countries—over the last few decades well correlates with the fall in bladder cancer mortality. Tobacco, however, can hardly account for a large proportion of the favorable trends registered in women over the last decade (Bosetti et al. 2013).

Part of the fall in women can be due to a better control of urinary tract infections, which have been related to increased risk of bladder cancer in case–control studies. This applies to men, too, though cystitis and other urinary tract infections are less frequent in men than in women. The relation between urinary tract infections and bladder cancer is however still open to discussion, since the results of cohort studies are inconsistent (Silverman et al. 2006). Dietary factors are also likely to play some role in bladder carcinogenesis, though the components of diet related to bladder cancer risk remain open to discussion (WCRF 2007).

With reference to occupational exposure, excesses bladder cancer risks have been reported among workers employed in aromatic amine manufacture, dyestuff manufacture and use, printing, rubber manufacture, in those exposed to polycyclic aromatic hydrocarbons and in truck drivers (Silverman et al. 2006) Occupational exposures were responsible for about 5 % of bladder cancer cases in high-resource countries, and probably for a larger proportion in selected areas. The control of occupational exposure to bladder carcinogens might have contributed to part of the decline in bladder cancer mortality over recent years, particularly in men.

The potential role of other factors, such as hair dyes or coffee drinking, on bladder cancer risk remains open to discussion.

A consistent relationship has been observed between use of phenacytic containing drugs and bladder cancer, with RR varying from two- to over sixfold. Cyclophosphamide, an alkylating agent which has been used to treat both malignant and non-malignant diseases has also been linked to bladder cancer. Studies based on cohorts of cancer patients indicate an increase in risk of approximately fivefold associated with cyclophosphamide therapy, with higher risks among heavily exposed subjects.

Schistosoma infection is prevalent throughout Africa and is associated with an increased risk of approximately fivefold. Cases associated with Schistosoma infection are mainly SqCC. They are responsible for an estimated 10 % of bladder cancer cases in the low-resource countries, and about 2 % of cases overall (Bedwani et al. 1998).

The enzymes, *N*-acetyl transferase 2 and glutathione-*S*-transferase are involved in the detoxification of various bladder carcinogens including arylamines. Variants in these genes may result in slow metabolization and in higher risk of bladder cancer, in particular among smokers (Garcia-Closas et al. 2005; Garcia-Closas et al. 2013). In addition, some rare genetic syndromes increase the risk for bladder cancer, including mutations of the retinoblastoma (RB1), Cowden disease, caused by mutations in PTEN, and Lynch syndrome (also known as hereditary non-polyposis colorectal cancer, or HNPCC), caused by mutations in mismatch repair genes.

Regarding prevention, avoidance of cigarette smoking is the most effective public health measure against bladder cancer. Approximately 50 % of bladder cancer cases are due to smoking, at least half of which could be prevented by smoking cessation among current smokers. Prevention of Schistosoma infection through avoidance of contaminated waters is important in endemic areas. No effective screening approach is available for bladder cancer.

4.13.2 Cancer of the Kidney

Worldwide, there were approximately 340,000 kidney cancers in 2012, two-thirds of which occurred in high-resource countries (Ferlay et al. 2013). The vast majority of cancers which arise in the renal parenchyma are adenocarcinomas, although nephroblastoma (Wilms' tumour) occurs in children. The highest incidences of renal cell cancers are observed in Central Europe and among Blacks in the US, with rates of approximately 20/100,000 in men and 10/100,000 in women. High rates are also observed in parts of Italy and Eastern Europe Conversely, rates up to ten times lower are reported in most Asian and African populations and some, but not all, South-American populations (Forman et al. 2013). Trends in incidence are different to interpret, since diagnosis of kidney cancer has largely improved through the use of echography and other imaging techniques. Mortality, however, has been declining over the last one or two decades in North America and Europe (Levi et al. 2004).

Tobacco smoking is the single best recognised risk factor for kidney cancer, and particularly for renal pelvis neoplasms, the RR being around 2 for smokers, with a proportional attributable risk of about one-third of cancers in men and 10 % in women in high-resource countries (McLaughlin et al. 2006). Thus, the decline in smoking prevalence in men over the last few decades in most high-resource countries may explain, at least in part, the decline in kidney cancer rates. Tobacco, however, cannot account for the trends observed in women.

Obesity, the second best recognised risk factor for kidney cancer (WCRF 2007), accounted for >20 % of cases in the USA. Dietary factors may play some role, but their influence on renal carcinogenesis remains unclear (WCRF 2007). Exposure to occupational carcinogens may play a role, although the impact of occupational exposures on kidney cancer risk remains unquantified (McLaughlin et al. 2006). Likewise, better control of urinary tract infections may also influence kidney cancer risk.

A history of hypertension has been linked to kidney cancer, although the strength of this relationship is greatly reduced after adjustment for use of diuretics and other anti-hypertensive drugs. These findings suggest that use of medications may be the primary risk factor and not hypertension per se. Both diuretic and non-diuretic anti-hypertensive medications have been linked to kidney cancer, with supportive evidence from animal studies. However, separating out whether the real risk is due to the hypertensive state or due to antihypertensive medication has not so far been possible. Whichever of the two is the real risk factor, it is likely to account for a substantial proportion of cases.

The main avoidable causes of kidney cancer are cigarette smoking and excess body weight, which together account for up to a third of all cases. Primary prevention in reducing cigarette smoking and obesity are therefore the clearest strategies for reducing the incidence of the disease. An undefined proportion of cases are also likely to be related to hypertension, which however is strongly related to overweight and obesity. Familial, and hence likely genetic factors, may account for 3–5 % of cancers.

4.13.3 Cancer of Renal Pelvis and Ureter

Renal pelvis and ureter cancers are mainly transitional cell carcinomas as opposed to adenocarcinomas of the kidney. Renal pelvis cancers occur with approximately 10 % the frequency of renal cell cancers and ureter cancers with a frequency of approximately 5 %. For both sites, high rates are observed in parts of Europe including northern Italy, Switzerland, the Czech Republic and Poland, as well as Australia and the USA. In the USA, rates are higher among Whites than Blacks, in contrast to the incidence of kidney cancer (Parkin et al. 2002). The male-to-female ratio is approximately 2–1.

The main risk factor for renal pelvis and ureter cancers is cigarette smoking, with up to fivefold increased risk for smokers compared to non-smokers (McLaughlin et al. 2006). The attributable proportion of renal pelvis and ureter cancers due to cigarette smoking has been estimated to be as high as 80 % among men and 40 % among women.

Exposure to aristolochic acids, a family of compounds found in the *Aristolochia* genus of plants, many of which are used in herbal remedies used in China and other countries, has been shown to caused a progressive interstitial renal fibrosis called aristolochic acid nephropathy. This disease, including its form called Balkan epidemic nephropathy, is associated with a very high risk of cancer of the renal pelvis and the ureter (Gokmen et al. 2013). Endemic areas include the Balkan countries and Taiwan, but cases of aristolochic acid-related urothelial cancer have been reported from many other countries, including Belgium, other Western European countries, China, and the United States. Although the use of medical remedies containing *Aristolochia* spp. has been forbidden in many countries, it is likely that exposure continues in many Asian countries where these plants are used as folk remedies.

A consistent relationship was also observed between use of phenacytin containing drugs and cancer of the renal pelvis. Because of concern of nephropathy linked to phenacetin use, it has been removed from analgesics in most countries, starting in the late 1960s.

Because of the high proportion of renal pelvic and ureter tumours caused by cigarette smoking, especially current smoking, encouraging current smokers to give up is likely to result in a substantial reduction in the number of cases.

4.14 Cancer of the Nervous Organs

4.14.1 Cancer of the Eye

Neoplasms of the eye are rare: the incidence is below 1/100,000 in all regions of the world, with the exception of Central and Southern Africa and some regions of South America (Ferlay et al. 2010b; Forman et al. 2013). The main histological types are SqCC, arising from the conjunctiva, RB, which arises in children and is relatively common in Africa, and uveal melanoma, which is the main adult type outside Africa. Solar radiation is a cause of conjunctiva carcinoma and uveal melanoma. About 50 % of cases of RB are caused by an inherited mutation in the Rb gene.

4.14.2 Cancer of the Nervous System

Over 90 % of nervous system neoplasms arise from the brain, the cranial nerves and the cranial meninges. Data on the descriptive epidemiology of neoplasms of the nervous system are difficult to interpret, because of inconsistent inclusion of benign tumours in different series of cases.

Gliomas arise from the glial cells and are classified pathologically as astrocytomas (low-grade) and glioblastomas (high-grade). They represent 40–60 % of primary tumours of the brain, are predominantly malignant, and are more common in men. Meningiomas arise from the cranial meninges and represent 20–35 % of brain neoplasms, while schwannomas (or neurilemomas) arise from the Schwann cells of the nerve sheath (mainly of the eight cranial—acoustic—nerve) and represent 5–10 % of all brain neoplasms. These two latter types are mainly benign. Rare types of nervous system neoplasms include pituitary adenomas, childhood primary neuroectodermal tumours (also called medulloblastoma), and tumours of the spine and the peripheral nerves.

The estimated number of cases of brain and nervous system care in 2008 was about 240,000 (85,000 in high income, 155,000 middle and low middle income countries) and the estimated number of deaths was about 80,000 (30 high, 50 low and middle income countries) (Ferlay et al. 2010a)).

The incidence of brain tumours is slightly higher in men than in women; the male-to-female ratio is approximately 1.3 for gliomas and 0.6 for meningiomas. There is a geographical variability in the incidence of brain neoplasms; rates in men are above 6/100,000 in most countries from the Americas, Europe and Oceania, and in the range 2–3/100,000 in Africa and Asia. Part of this variation, however, can be attributed to different diagnostic accuracy in various areas of the world. In the USA, rates of gliomas are 30–50 % higher in Whites than in other ethnic groups, while rates of meningiomas are slightly higher in Blacks (Forman et al. 2013). The incidence of gliomas tends to be higher among people from high socio-economic groups.

During the past decades, incidence and mortality from brain tumours have increased in most high-income countries, but have recently tended to level off. Thus, apparent upward trends and differences in the descriptive epidemiology of brain cancer, including time trends, can be partially or largely attributed to variations in diagnostic and reporting procedures.

Ionizing radiation is the only established non-genetic risk factor for brain tumours (Preston-Martin et al. 2006). It causes all three major types of central nervous system tumours, but the association is stronger for meningioma and schwannoma than for glioma. The evidence comes mainly from studies of atomic bomb survivors and of patients given X-ray therapy in the head and neck region. Head trauma has been suggested as a risk factor for meningioma, and acoustic trauma (as in the case of jobs with exposure to loud noise) as a risk factor for acoustic schwannoma, but the association can be partly or largely due to reporting bias. *N*-nitroso compounds, in particular nitrosoureas, are potent experimental brain carcinogens, but the evidence of an aetiological role in humans is inconclusive. Several other lifestyle (e.g., tobacco smoking), environmental (e.g., occupational exposures) and medical (e.g., allergic conditions) factors have been suggested to play an etiological role in brain cancer, but the evidence in not sufficient to draw any conclusion. Alcohol drinking does not appear to be associated with adult brain cancer, though a potential effect of high doses remain open to discussion (Galeone et al. 2013).

Tumours of the central nervous system occur frequently in rare congenital syndromes, such as neurofibromatosis types 1 and 2, von Hippel–Lindau syndrome and Li–Fraumeni syndrome.

The very limited knowledge about the aetiology of tumours of the central nervous system offers scarce resources for an effective preventive strategy.

4.15 Cancer of Endocrine Glands

4.15.1 Thyroid Cancer

An estimated 230,000 new cases of thyroid cancer occurred in 2008 among women, and 70,000 among men (Ferlay et al. 2013). In most areas of the world, the incidence among women is in the range 2–5/100,000, that in men is between 1 and 2/100,000. High-risk areas (incidence over 10/100,000 in women) include South and North America, Italy in Europe, Japan and the Pacific islands (Forman et al. 2013). International comparisons, however, are complicated by possible differences in diagnostic procedures. The most common thyroid neoplasm (50–80 % of the total) is papillary carcinoma, followed by follicular (10–40 %) and medullary carcinoma (5–15 %).

Survival from thyroid cancer, particularly for papillary carcinoma in the young, is very good (over 85 % five-year survival rate in Europe or North America), resulting in low mortality rates (below 1.2/100,000 in women and 0.6/100,000 in men in most areas of the world).

In most countries, incidence rates have been stable or have been slowly increasing during the last decades; mortality rates have steadily declined, likely because of improved diagnosis, management at treatment.

Ionizing radiation, particularly in young childhood is the main established risk factor for thyroid cancer (Ron and Schneider 2006). The pooled analysis of studies of individuals irradiated in childhood for medical conditions and atomic bomb survivors resulted in a summary excess RR of 7.7 per Gy, and an excess absolute risk of 4.4 per 10,000 person-years Gy. Several studies have been published on adults exposed to ^{131}I for medical purposes. Although those studies suggest an increased risk, their interpretation is complicated by the fact that some of these patients were treated because of thyroid diseases. ^{131}I was the main exposure resulting from the accident of the Chernobyl nuclear reactor in 1986: since then, an increased incidence of thyroid cancer has been reported among children living in the contaminated areas of Belarus and Ukraine. Studies of occupational exposure to low-level ionizing radiation, typically in the nuclear industry, have failed to show an increased incidence of thyroid cancer.

An association between thyroid cancer and a history of benign thyroid diseases has been consistently reported, although the strengths of these associations have varied across studies up to 4–5-fold. Because thyroid cancer incidence rates in women are 2–3 times higher than those in men, some studies in various geographic areas have focused on women in an attempt to identify hormonal factors that might explain this excess. However, findings related to menstrual and reproductive factors, as well as to exogenous hormone use, have been inconsistent.

In a pooled analysis (Franceschi et al. 1999), goiter and benign nodules/adenomas were the strongest risk factors for thyroid cancer apart from radiation in childhood. Elevated risk was observed for men and women and in relation to both major histologic types. The excess risk was greatest within 2–4 years prior to thyroid cancer diagnosis, but an elevated RR was present 10 years or more before cancer. Prior hyperthyroidism was related to a small, non-significant increase that was reduced after allowance for a history of goiter. A history of hypothyroidism was not associated with cancer risk.

Elevated levels of thyroid-stimulating hormones are associated with thyroid growth and possibly thyroid cancer. The evidence of an association between iodine deficiency (and presence of endemic goiter) and thyroid cancer is equivocal: studies from Central and Southern Europe support such an association, which however was not confirmed in studies from Northern Europe and North America. It is possible that iodine deficiency increases the risk of follicular thyroid cancer, while the papillary type is linked to iodine-rich diet.

Among dietary factors, pooled analyses focused mainly on fish/seafood (Bosetti et al. 2001) and cruciferous and other vegetables (Bosetti et al. 2002). Fish was not associated with thyroid cancer risk in all studies combined, but there was a suggestion of reduced risk in endemic goiter areas. However, high levels of fish consumption did not appreciably increase risk in iodine-rich areas, and fish consumption was inversely related to thyroid cancer risk in endemic goiter areas. Cruciferous vegetables, which contain goitrogenic substances as well as several constituents which can inhibit carcinogenesis, were weakly and inconsistently related to reduced risk of thyroid cancer (Dal Maso et al. 2009).

There is a strong genetic component for medullary carcinoma: about 20 % of these neoplasms are associated with an autosomal dominant gene with penetrance close to 100 % (Negri et al. 2002). It can also be associated with other endocrine neoplasms within the multiple endocrine neoplasia syndromes. Familial factors play a role in papillary carcinoma, too. Among the genes associated with thyroid cancer, there are the ret proto-oncogene (for papillary and medullary carcinomas) and the APC gene for papillary carcinoma.

The prospects for prevention of thyroid cancer are made complex by the limited understanding of its aetiology, with the exception of relatively rare high-risk conditions, such as childhood exposure to ionizing radiation.

Early diagnosis has been widely adopted, through new imaging techniques, but its impact on thyroid cancer mortality remains unquantified.

4.15.2 Cancer of Other Endocrine Glands

Malignant neoplasms of endocrine glands other than the thyroid are rare in most populations. The incidence rates range between 0.1 and 1/100,000 persons (Forman et al. 2013). About two-thirds of these neoplasms arise from the adrenal gland. About one-third of these tumours are carcinomas, and the remaining proportion shows different histological types.

Genetic susceptibility plays a relatively important role for this group of neoplasms: in particular, adrenocortical carcinoma is found in cases of Li–Fraumeni syndrome, and malignant pheochromocytoma is found in the multiple endocrine neoplasia type 2 and the von Hippel–Lindau syndromes. Tobacco smoking has been associated with an increased risk of adrenal cancer in a few studies. The evidence for a carcinogenic role of other factors is inconclusive.

4.16 Neoplasms of the Lymphatic and Haematopoietic Organs

The term lymphoma encompasses a diverse group of neoplasms which originate from the cells of the lymphopoietic system. Traditionally, two main groups of lymphomas have been distinguished including HL, characterized by large polynuclear cells named after Reed and Sternberg, and a diverse group of other neoplasms, defined as non-Hodgkin's lymphomas (NHL). The complexity of lymphomas is reflected by the various classifications that have been used to separate different subtypes. The most recent World Health Organisation (WHO) classification system (Jaffe et al. 2008) represents an effort to reach a consensus to allocate all lymphoma cases in clear categories. Neoplasms are divided in two large groups: those originating from mature B-cells, including multiple myeloma, B-cell acute lymphoblastic leukaemia, Burkitt's lymphoma and HL, and those originating from mature T- and NK-cells. Each group is then subdivided into more than 20 different clinicopathological entities. Given that this classification has only been in use for a number of years, it is still necessary to discuss the characteristics of lymphomas and leukaemias under the traditional entities.

4.16.1 Hodgkin Lymphoma

Hodgkin lymphoma accounts for about 65,000 cases and 25,000 deaths worldwide in 2012 (Ferlay et al. 2013). The incidence of Hodgkin Lymphoma (HL) varies from low-incidence populations, with rates lower than 1/100,000, including areas of Southern and Eastern Asia and of Sub-Saharan Africa, to high-incidence populations, with rates in the order of 3/100,000 found in the USA and some European countries, as well as in Israeli Jews (Forman et al. 2013). The incidence in men is consistently higher than in women with a ratio of between 1.5 and 2. The incidence has been relatively stable over time and may even be declining. The age of onset of HL shows a bimodal distribution in high-resource populations with a first peak between age 15 and 35 and a second peak after the age of 60. In low-income countries the first peak tends to be observed during childhood. This bimodal distribution suggests that the HL includes at least two different entities.

Mortality from Hodgkin's lymphomas has substantially decreased since the 1970s in North America, wester Europe and Japan, due to improved treatment, but the falls have been later in other areas of the world, including Central and Eastern Europe and Latin America. Over recent years, however, Argentina and Brazil—but not eastern Europe—have reached mortality rates comparable to high income countries (Chatenoud et al. 2013).

Viral infections play an important role in the aetiology of HL (Mueller and Grufferman 2006). Its onset may be related to decreased or delayed exposure to infectious agents during childhood, as indicated by its association with having fewer siblings, living in single family houses, and early birth order.

Infection with EBV is associated with the majority of HL cases. EBV is ubiquitous throughout the world with 80–100 % of individuals being infected by age 30 (IARC 1997). In low-resource countries infection occurs earlier in life, whereas in high-resource countries infection is often delayed until adolescence. EBV genome is present in about 50 % of the lymphoma cells of cases, and another EBV-related condition, infectious mononucleosis, is associated with a moderately elevated risk of development of HL. Sero-epidemiological studies indicate that patients with HL can be distinguished by an altered antibody profile to EBV.

A type 2 immune environment (predominance of Th2 cytokines and chemokines, and in particular of interleukin 13) is present in HL, but its etiological role is unclear. Patients suffering from immunodeficiencies or autoimmune diseases are at increased risk of HL. A link between HL and lifestyle and environmental (e.g., occupation) factors has not been established.

HL patients have an increased familial risk of HL and NHL; this evidence is supported by the results of genomewide analyses, which showed a role of loci in the major histocompatibility complex region (Urayama et al. 2012).

4.16.2 Non-Hodgkin Lymphoma

In 2012, non Hodgkin lymphomas accounts for about 385,000 cases and 200,000 deaths worldwide (Ferlay et al. 2013). The incidence of NHL is higher than the incidence of HL. Rates of over 15/100,000 in men and 10/100,000 in women are reported from the USA, Australia, Western Europe, and from Israel, while low rates of less than 5/100,000 are reported from Southern and Eastern Asia and sub-Saharan Africa (Parkin et al. 2002). Men have a 1.5–2-fold higher incidence than women. There is a strong geographical variation for some lymphoma subgroups. For example, Burkitt's lymphoma is common among children in eastern Africa, and rates of adult T-cell leukaemia/lymphoma are increased in Japan and parts of Africa. The trend by age of NHL, on the other hand, shows a steady increase with age in most populations. Exceptions are the populations in which a specific type of lymphoma predominates, such as Burkitt's lymphoma in children.

An increase in the incidence of NHL has been observed in most high-resource countries until the end of the twentieth century. The rate of increase was approximately 4 % per year in most populations. In the last decade, however, the increase has ceased. The reasons for the increase in NHL incidence have been widely discussed and it is possible that improvement in diagnostic procedures explains part of it, in particular in the elderly. However, it is now accepted that the trend also reflected a real increase in the number of cases, the causes of which are not known.

The knowledge of potential risk factors for NHL is limited (Hartge et al. 2006). However, there is strong evidence that altered immunological function, either immunostimulation or immuno-suppression, entails an increased risk of NHL. For example, immunosuppressed renal transplant patients have a risk 30 times higher for developing NHL compared to the general population. Lymphomas that develop in immunosuppressed patients share common characteristics. They are generally high-grade B-cell lymphomas and are more likely to be extranodal and of worse prognosis. Lymphomas have also been reported for a variety of other conditions which are either auto-immune in nature, or require immunosuppressive treatment, including Sjögren's syndrome and systemic lupus erithematosous.

Infectious agents associated with NHL include HIV, human T-cell lymphotropic virus 1 EBV and HCV. Human T-cell lymphotropic virus 2, and human herpes viruses 6 and 8 have also been linked to the development of NHL. In addition, infection with *Helicobacter pylori* is a risk factor for gastric lymphoma.

EBV is particularly prominent in lymphomas developing in immunosuppressed patients, and also in Burkitt's lymphomas. The relationship with other forms of lymphoma is, however, unclear. Regarding HIV, NHL is 60 times more frequent among patients with AIDS than in the general population (IARC 1996). About 3 % of the patients with AIDS developed a NHL, which represents a small contribution to the overall incidence of NHL, except in populations with a high HIV prevalence such as regions of sub-Saharan Africa. AIDS-related lymphomas tend to be high-grade B-cell lymphomas.

Human T-cell lymphotropic virus 1, and possibly human T-cell lymphotropic virus 2, appear to be associated with the rare adult T-cell leukaemia/lymphoma, a disease entity with strong geographical clustering in Japan, the Caribbean and parts of Africa. Transmission of the human T-cell lymphotropic virus is similar to that of HIV, involving vertical (mother-to-child) transmission, sexual contact or blood transfusion.

A familial aggregation is present for NHL: the risk of the disease among first-degree relatives of cases has been reported in the order of 1.5–4. However, the risk seems higher for sibs of the same sex, suggesting a role of shared environmental factors rather than genetics. Highly penetrant genetic predisposition to lymphomas is not very common but include ataxia telangiectasia, Wiskott–Aldrich syndrome and hypogammaglobulinemia. Approximately 25 % of the patients with rare forms of genetic immunodeficiency will develop a lymphoma.

The increasing recreational exposure to ultraviolet radiation in some populations and the decrease in the atmospheric ozone layer have been related to the observed increase in the incidence of NHL, but this hypothesis has not been supported by analytical studies, which, if anything, showed a decreased risk of NHL for high UV exposure (Armstrong and Kricker 2007).

Exposure to pesticides has been associated to NHL risk in studies conducted both on manufacturing workers and applicators in agriculture. The results, however, are not very compelling, with the possible exception of phenoxy herbicides and chlorophenols. This effect might be due to contamination with dioxin. Farming as an occupation has also been weakly associated with NHL risk. Organic solvents represent another group of chemicals whose association with NHL risk has been widely investigated, without conclusive findings.

4.16.3 Multiple Myeloma

In 2012, multiple myeloma occurred for about 114,000 cases worldwide, and for 90,000 deaths (Ferlay et al. 2013).

Multiple myeloma is a malignancy of the plasma cells with a variable manifestation. High-incidence areas of around 4/100,000 include North America, Western Europe and Oceania. Low rates of around 1–2/100,000 are reported in most of Asia, although part of this may be due to under-diagnosis. Within the USA, Blacks have approximately double the incidence rate of Whites, with the incidence approaching 10/100,000 in some areas (Forman et al. 2013). Whether this increase among American Blacks is due to genetic or to environmental effects is unknown. In most populations incidence rates are higher in men although the ratio is usually less than 2. Multiple myeloma is a disease of the elderly, and rates are very low among young adults. It also appears that the incidence of myeloma increased until the mid-1990s, although these trends are difficult to judge and may be due to diagnostic artefacts.

The only established risk factor for multiple myeloma is monoclonal gammopathy of unknown significance, an asymptomatic non-malignant disorder involving proliferation of plasma cells. The increased risk associated with monoclonal gammopathy of unknown significance (MGUS) appears to be in the order of tenfold, although the lifetime absolute risk is still relatively low (<5 %). The causes of MGUS are largely unknown. Other conditions have also been reported to be associated with myeloma including rheumatoid arthritis and allergies, although the evidence is inconclusive.

Ionizing radiation is associated with myeloma risk. Occupational groups which have been reported to have higher myeloma rates include painters and farmers, which might be due to exposure to benzene, animal pathogens or pesticides, although results are inconsistent.

4.16.4 Leukaemias

In 2012, there were about 350,000 cases of leukemias worldwide, and 265,000 deaths from leukemia (Ferlay et al. 2013). Leukaemias arise in one of the types of white blood cells. They may arise in lymphoblasts, which are lymphoid cells in the early stage of development, resulting in a rapid onset illness termed acute lymphoblastic leukaemia. Alternatively, when the neoplasm involves mature cells, it is termed chronic lymphocytic leukaemia and is usually more sedate. In the WHO classification (Jaffe et al. 2008), acute and chronic lymphocytic leukemia are part of NHL. Leukaemias may also be granulocytic in origin, occurring in either young myeloblastic cells resulting in acute myeloid leukaemia, or in the mature granulocytes resulting in chronic myeloid leukaemia. There also exist several rarer varieties including monocytic and hairy cell leukaemias.

Acute lymphoblastic leukaemia is the most common childhood cancer, while over 80 % of lymphoid leukaemias occurring in adulthood are chronic lymphocytic leukaemia. Incidence rates for chronic lymphocytic leukaemia are difficult to interpret because it is often diagnosed incidentally, or in the course of evaluating other conditions. Differences in medical care may therefore substantially bias incidence data. Bearing this possible ascertainment bias in mind, the highest rates of lymphoid leukaemias are observed in areas of Canada, the USA, Western Europe and Oceania, and are lowest ones in South America the Caribbean, Asia and Africa. Rates tend to be lower in females although the ratio is usually less than 2. Some increases in leukaemia over time have been reported although the extent to which these represent real increases in incidence is unclear. Some increasing incidence trends have been reported for both chronic myeloid leukaemia and acute myeloid leukaemia, although these are not consistent and may simply reflect changes in diagnostic practices.

Although the cause of most leukaemias is not known, there is consistent evidence for three factors, namely ionizing radiation, alkylating agents used in chemotherapy, and occupational benzene exposure (Linet et al. 2007). Leukaemia was the first cancer to be linked to ionizing radiation after the atomic bombings in Hiroshima and Nagasaki, and excesses have been observed for acute lymphoblastic leukaemia, acute myeloid leukaemia and chronic myeloid leukaemia, but not for chronic lymphocytic leukaemia. Cohorts of patients who have received radiotherapy for both malignant and non-malignant conditions have also been found to be at an increased risk of leukaemia, usually myeloid. Whether there is any increased risk of leukaemia from other sources, including low-level diagnostic radiation, occupational exposure in the nuclear industry for workers and their offspring, or nuclear test explosions, is more contentious. Part of the problem lies in extrapolating from high acute doses experienced in particular circumstances like atomic bombing , to small or chronic exposures in other instances. There is no consistent evidence that exposure to electromagnetic fields is associated with leukaemia risk.

Some leukaemias are also related to, or induced by therapy for a prior malignancy, most notably HL. Such patients have a 20–40-fold increased risk of leukaemia, most of which are acute myeloid leukaemia. The risk appears to be related to chemotherapy including alkylating agents (in particular Mission Oriented Protective Posture (MOPP) combination therapy). The effect is greater when patients are treated with both chemotherapy and radiotherapy, although whether an independent effect exists for radiotherapy is unclear. Other chemotherapy regimes which appear to be associated to acute myeloid leukaemia are those which contain the epipodophyllotoxin drugs teniposide and etoposide.

Occupational benzene exposure is also a recognized cause of acute myeloid leukaemi (AML). An increased risk of between three- and fivefold has been observed in several occupational cohorts of workers exposure to high levels of benzene, as it occurred in the past in shoe manufacturing, rubber manufacturing and printing. This was frequently preceded by aplastic anemia. The role of low dose exposure on AML—and other lymphoid neoplasms—remains unquantified. Tobacco smoking is a cause of acute myeloid leukemia, possibly because of the relatively high levels of benzene present in the smoke.

4.16.5 Prevention of Lymphoid Neoplasms

The limited knowledge of the causes of lymphatic and haematopoietic neoplasms limits the opportunity for prevention. Avoidance of known risk factors (e.g., unnecessary radiation exposure, benzene) is likely to result in the prevention of a small proportion of these neoplasms in most populations.

4.17 Childhood and Adolescence Cancers

Acute lymphoblastic leukemia and acute myeloid leukemia account for the large majority of childhood leukemias, and hence for over 50 % of all childhood cancers in most population.

Several chromosomal rearrangements are present in childhood leukemia, and Down syndrome and ataxia-telangiectasia appreciably increase the risk of both types of leukemia. In utero diagnostic radiotherapy was associated to the risk of both types of childhood leukemia, but the doses have substantially decreased over the last few decades, and consequently the public health implications are now minor. Childhood leukemia is directly related to high socioeconomic status, and both types of leukemias have been related to a rare and late response to infection, though the pathogenic agent has and not been established. The role of other risk factors, including non ionising radiation, maternal smoking, paternal occupation, exposure to benzene or pesticides remains unclear (Ross and Spector 2006).

Central nervous system cancers of various histologic types account for about one in six childhood cancers. They have been associated to nitrosamines, polyoma viruses and pesticides, but the evidence is not conclusive and there is therefore no known cause. Except for astrocitoma survival is relatively lower than for most other childhood cancers.

HL in children has also been related to higher socioeconomics status, and shows a genetic predisposition. Its prognosis has substantially improved over the last few decades, and now survival is over 90 % in high-income countries.

Most NHL in children are high grade tumours, including lymphoblastic lymphoma, Burkitt lymphoma and anaplastic lymphoma. Burkitt lymphoma accounts from most cases diagnosed in Africa, and is related to EBV infection. Apart from genetic factors (ataxia-telangiectasia, Wiscott–Aldrich syndrome), no other risk factor is known.

Other types of childhood cancer include soft tissue sarcoma, neuroblastoma, renal cell cancers (Wilms tumor), bone tumors (osteosarcoma, Ewing sarcoma) germ cell cancers, hepatoblastoma and retinoblastoma RB. The latter is related to the RB gene.

Despite progress over recent years, the advancements in treatment were later and inadequate in Eastern Europe in Latin America, and in most low and middle income countries. Mortality from all childhood cancer over recent years was 2–4/100,000 boys and 1.5–3/100,000 girls in North America, most western Europe, and Japan, but 5–6/100,000 boys and 3.5–5.5 girls in most central and eastern Europe and Latin America. Similar proportional differentials were observed in childhood leukemias (Chatenoud et al. 2010; Bosetti et al. 2012d).

At ages 15–19 years, a different proportional composition of various neoplasms is observed, with a rise of testicular cancer in boys, germ cell ovarian neoplasms in girls and, mostly, bone cancer in both genders combined. Nonetheless, mortality from all neoplasms, as well as from leukaemias, declined by over 50 % since the late 1960s in North America at in Western Europe, while in Eastern Europe and in other low and middle income areas of the world some decline in cancer mortality was observed only during the last two decades—as for childhood cancers—again reflecting the delayed and inadequate adoption of efficacious treatment for various cancers. This is reflected also within each neoplasm, including the ones most amenable to treatment, such as HL or leukaemia, and calls for urgent widespread adoption of modern and integrated treatment for childhood and adolescent cancers worldwide.

The decline in cancer mortality at age 15–19, moreover, was smaller than at age 10–14, calling for the importance of integrated cancer management in this age group, too.

Chapter 5
Overview of the Major Causes of Human Cancer

Keywords Tobacco smoking • Dietary factors • Obesity • Physical exercise • Alcohol drinking • Infectious agents • Pollution • Ionizing radiation • Non-ionizing radiation • Genetic factors

5.1 Tobacco Smoking

Tobacco smoking is the main single cause of human cancer worldwide (IARC 2004) and the largest cause of death and disease. It is the key cause of lung cancer, and a major cause of cancers of the oral cavity, pharynx, nasal cavity, larynx, oesophagus, stomach, pancreas, uterine cervix, kidney and bladder, as well as of myeloid leukemia. In high-resource countries, tobacco smoking causes approximately 30 % of all human cancers (Doll and Peto 2005). In many medium- and low-income countries, the burden of tobacco-related cancer is still lower, given the relatively recent start of the epidemics of smoking, which will however result in a greater numbers of cancer in the future, in the absence of adequate intervention to control tobacco.

A benefit of quitting tobacco smoking in adulthood has been shown for all major cancers causally associated with the habit. Smokers who stop around age 50 avoid over 50 % of overall excess mortality from all causes (Doll et al. 2004; Jha et al. 2013; Pirie et al. 2013), from lung cancers (Peto et al. 2000) and well as from other tobacco-related cancers (Bosetti et al. 2008a), and those who stop around age 40 or earlier avoid most of their tobacco-related cancer risk.

This emphasizes the need to devise anti-smoking strategies that address avoidance of the habit among the young, as well as reduction of smoking and quitting among adults. In fact, the decline in tobacco consumption that has taken place during the last half century among men in North America and several European countries, and which has resulted in decreased incidence of and mortality from lung cancer (La Vecchia et al. 2010; Bosetti et al. 2012c; Malvezzi et al. 2013b), was caused primarily by quitting at middle age. The great challenge for the control of

P. Boffetta et al., *A Quick Guide to Cancer Epidemiology*, SpringerBriefs in Cancer Research, DOI 10.1007/978-3-319-05068-3_5,

tobacco-related cancer, however, lies today in middle and low-income countries, in particular in China and the other Asian countries: the largest increase in tobacco-related cancers has been forecasted in this region of the world (Peto et al. 1999). The control of tobacco related cancers in the first half of this century is essentially due to stopping in middle age, since diseases and deaths in adolescents who stand now with occur in the second half of the century. Despite growing efforts from medical and public health institutions and the growing involvement of non-governmental organizations, the fight against the spread of tobacco smoking among women and in middle low-income countries remains the biggest and most difficult challenge of cancer prevention in the next decades. In 2008 the WHO has established the MPOWER policy package highlighting priority interventions towards tobacco control (Song et al. 2013). The evidence base for the effect of the MPOWER recommendations is still limited, though the prevalence of tobacco smoking has declined across the WHO region. Modelling suggests, however, that it will be difficult to achieve rates below 10 % within a 20-year time horizon (Mendez et al. 2013).

Use of smokeless tobacco products has been associated with increased risk of cancer of the head and neck and the pancreas (IARC 2004), though the data remain open to discussion (Bertuccio et al. 2011). Chewing of tobacco-containing products is particularly prevalent in Southern Asia, where it represents a major cause of oral and pharyngeal cancer.

5.2 Dietary Factors

The role of dietary factors in causing human cancer remains largely obscure. For no dietary factor other than alcohol (see Sect. 4.4) and aflatoxin (a carcinogen produced by some fungi in certain tropical areas) there is sufficient evidence of an increased or decreased risk of cancer. In particular, a role of intake of fat in determining breast and colorectal cancer risk has not been confirmed by recent meta-analyses (Alexander et al. 2010; Liu et al. 2011). A high intake of red and processed meat, instead of, has been associated with an increased risk of colorectal cancer in a meta-analysis of prospective studies (Chan et al. 2011), and a protective effect has been reported for fish intake (Wu et al. 2012), milk and total dairy products (Aune et al. 2012), and magnesium intake (Chen et al. 2012).

On the basis of available data, the World Cancer Research Foundation 2007 (WCRF 2007) on animal food intake recommends as public health goal that the population average consumption of red meat to be no more than 300 g (11 oz) a week, very little if any of which to be processed.

Concerning vegetable intake, the World Cancer Research Foundation 2007 report (WCRF 2007) gave probable evidence of risk reduction with cancers of the mouth and pharynx, larynx, esophagus and stomach, and limited evidence for nasopharynx, lung, colorectum, ovarium and endometrium. With reference to fruit, it gave probable evidence of risk reduction for mouth and pharynx, larynx, esophagus, lung and stomach, and limited for nasopharynx, pancreas, liver and colorectum.

A number of vitamins and other micronutrients or food components (including carotenoids, lycopene and flavonoids) showed an inverse relation with cancer risk. With reference to flavonoids, there are suggestions for a protective role of flavanones on upper aerodigestive tract, proanthocyanidins on gastric cancer, flavonols and proanthocyanidins on colorectal, flavonols and flavones on breast, and isoflavones on ovarian cancers (Pelucchi et al. 2009).

There is evidence suggestive lack of cancer-preventive activity for preformed vitamin A (IARC 1998b) and for ß-carotene when used at high doses (IARC 1998a), and a lack of evidence of increased cancer risk associated with vitamin D status (IARC 2008). Systematic reviews have concluded that nutritional factors may be responsible for about one-fourth of human cancers in high-resource countries, although, because of the limitations of the current understanding of the precise role of diet in human cancer, the proportion of cancers known to be avoidable in practicable ways is much smaller (Doll and Peto 2005). The only justified dietary recommendation for cancer prevention is to reduce total caloric intake, which would contribute to a decrease in obesity, an established risk factor for human cancer (see Sect. 4.3).

5.3 Obesity and Physical Exercise

There is sufficient evidence for a cancer preventive effect of avoidance of weight gain, based on a decreased risk of cancers of the colon, gallbladder, post-menopausal breast, endometrium, kidney and esophagus (adenocarcinoma) (IARC 2002). The recommendation number one of the World Cancer Research Foundation 2007 report (WCRF 2007) suggest to "be as lean as possible within the normal range of body weight".

It is likely that obesity exerts a carcinogenic effect in conjunction with other factors such as insulin resistance, low physical activity and menopausal status. The magnitude of the excess risk is not very high (for most cancers the RR ranges between 1.5 and 2 for body weight higher than 35 % above the ideal weight). Estimates of the proportion of cancers attributable to overweight and obesity in Europe range from 2 % (Doll and Peto 2005) to 5 % (Bergstrom et al. 2001). However, this figure is likely to larger in North American, where the prevalence of overweight and obesity is higher.

Increasing physical activity should be part of any comprehensive cancer prevention strategy. Increased workplace or recreational physical activity decreased the risk of colon and breast cancers and that of endometrial and prostate cancers (IARC 2002). The RR of colon and breast cancers for regular versus no activity is in the order of 1.5–2. Worldwide, physical inactivity (defined as do not engage any brisk walking for at least 30 min every day), causes 10 % (5.6–14.1) of breast cancer, and 10 % (5.7–13.8) of colon cancer cases (Lee et al. 2012).

5.4 Alcohol Drinking

Alcohol drinking increases the risk of cancers of the oral cavity, pharynx, larynx, oesophagus and liver, colorectum and female breast (Baan et al. 2007). For all cancer sites, risk is a function of the amount of alcohol consumed. Alcohol drinking and tobacco smoking show an interactive effect on the risk of cancers of the head and neck (see Fig. 4.1).

Heavy alcohol consumption (i.e., ≥4 drinks/day) is significantly associated with an about fivefold increased risk of oral and pharyngeal cancer and esophageal squamous cell carcinoma, 2.5-fold for laryngeal cancer, 50 % for colorectal and breast cancers, and 30 % for pancreatic cancer (Pelucchi et al. 2011) (Fig. 5.1). These estimates are based on a large number of epidemiological studies, and are generally consistent across strata of several covariates. The evidence suggests that at low doses of alcohol consumption (i.e., ≤1 drink/day) the risk is also increased by about 20 % for oral and pharyngeal cancer and 30 % for esophageal squamous cell carcinoma (Fig. 5.2). Thus, for these sites there is no evidence of a threshold effect. While consumption of less than three alcoholic drinks/week is not associated with an increased risk of breast cancer, an intake of 3–6 drinks/week might already yield a (small) increase in risk. On the other hand, intakes up to one drink/day are not associated to the risk of laryngeal, colorectal and pancreatic cancer (Bagnardi et al. 2013). The dose-risk relation between causal of alcohol drinking and the risk of selected neoplasm is given in Fig. 5.3.

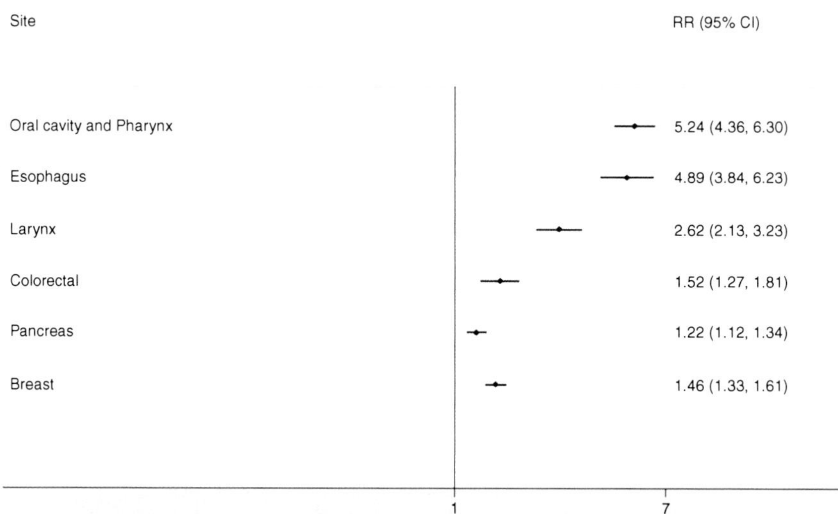

Fig. 5.1 Heavy alcohol drinking (Estimates for alcohol consumption of four or more drinks/day vs. non/occasional drinkers, except for pancreatic (i.e., ≥3 drinks/day vs. non/occasional drinkers) and breast (i.e., ≥45 g/day vs. non-drinkers) cancers.) and the risk of selected cancers (modified) (Pelucchi et al. 2011)

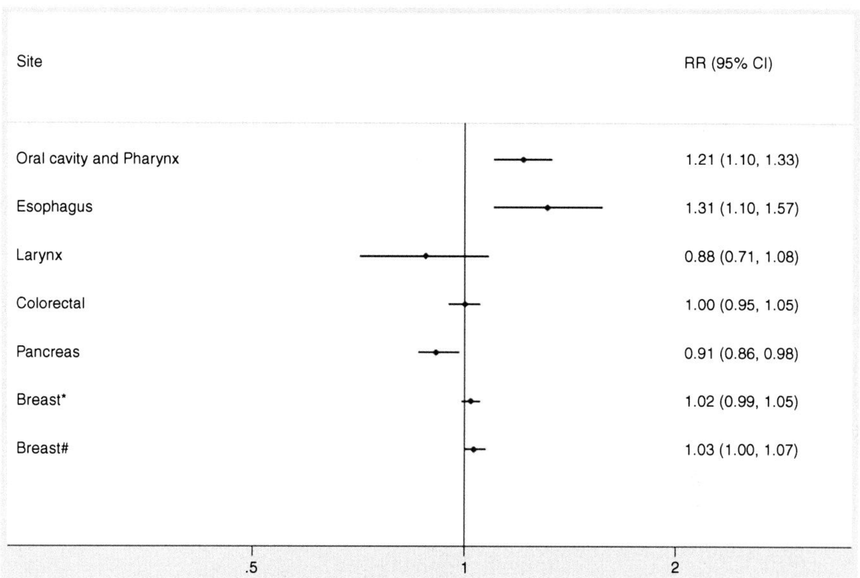

Fig. 5.2 Light alcohol drinking (Estimates for alcohol consumption of one or less drink/day vs. non/occasional drinkers, except for breast cancer.) and the risk of selected cancers (modified) (Pelucchi et al. 2011; Bagnardi et al. 2013). *Estimate for alcohol consumption of 14 or less g/day vs. non-drinkers. #Estimate for alcohol consumption of six or less drinks/week vs. non-drinkers

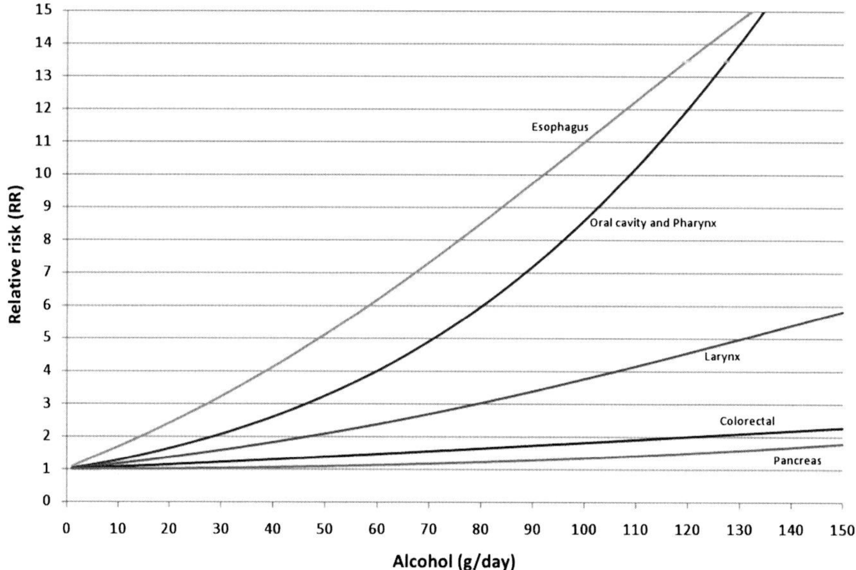

Fig. 5.3 Dose–response relation between alcohol drinking and the risk of selected cancers (modified) (Pelucchi et al. 2011)

The positive association between alcohol consumption and the risk of head and neck cancers is independent from tobacco exposure (Pelucchi et al. 2011). The global burden of cancer attributable to alcohol drinking has been estimated at 3.6 and 3.5 % of cancer deaths (Boffetta 2006), although this figure is higher in high-resource countries (e.g., the figure of 6 % has been proposed for United Kingdom (Doll and Peto 2005) , and 9 % in Central and Eastern Europe).

These included over 5 % of cancers and cancer deaths in men and about 1.5 % of cancers and cancer deaths in women. Restriction of alcohol drinking to the limits indicated by the European Code Against Cancer (Boyle et al. 2003) (20 g/day for men and 10 g/day for women) would avoid about 90 % of cancers and cancer deaths in men and over 50 % of cancers in women, i.e. about 330/360,000 cancer cases and about 200/220,000 cancer deaths. Avoidance, or moderation of alcohol consumption to two drinks/day in men and one drink/day in women is therefore a global public health priority.

5.5 Infectious Agents

There is growing evidence that chronic infection with some viruses, bacteria and parasites represents a major risk factor for human cancer, in particular in low-income countries. A number of infectious agents have been evaluated within the IARC Monograph programme (Table 5.1), and the evidence of a causal association has been classified as sufficient for several of them. A global burden of cancers attributable to infections in 2008 has been published in 2012 (de Martel et al. 2012). The population attributable fraction for infectious agents was 16.1 % in 2008, meaning that around two million new cancer cases were attributable to infections. HBV- and HCV-related liver cancer, HPV-related cervical cancer and *Helicobacter pylori*-related stomach cancer overall are responsible for 95 % of the total number of infection-related cancers. The estimate of the attributable fraction is higher in less developed countries than in high-resource countries (22.9 % of total cancer versus 7.4 %).

Use of safe, effective (and ideally cheap) vaccines represents the best preventive strategy for cancers caused by viruses, and HBV and HPV infection can be effectively prevented today. Chronic infection with *Helicobacter pylori* can be prevented by eradication treatment and sanitation measures, and changes in dietary practices (e.g., avoidance of raw fish) can prevent infection by carcinogenic parasites.

5.6 Occupation and Pollution

Approximately 40 occupational agents, groups of agents and mixtures have been classified as carcinogenic by IARC (Table 5.2). While some (e.g., bis-chloromethyl-ether) represent today a historic curiosity, exposure is still present for carcinogens

Table 5.1 Assessment of associations between infections and human cancer, from IARC Monographs as indicated

	Evidence[a]	Target organs[b]	IARC Monographs volume
Viruses			
Hepatitis B virus	S	Liver, bile duct (leukemia/ lymphoma)	59, 100B
Hepatitis C virus	S	Liver, bile duct, leukemia/ lymphoma	59, 100B
Hepatitis D virus	I	Liver	59
Human papillomavirus type 16	S	Cervix, vulva, vagina, penis, anus, oral cavity, tonsil, pharynx, (larynx)	64, 90, 100B
Human papillomavirus type 18	S	Cervix, (oral cavity), (penis), (anus), (vulva)	64, 90, 100B
Human papillomavirus types 31, 35, 39, 45, 51, 52, 56, 58, 59	S	Cervix	64, 90, 100B
Human papillomavirus type 33	S	Cervix, (Anus), (vulva)	64, 90, 100B
Human papillomavirus types 6, 11	I	(Larynx)	90, 100B
Human papillomavirus types 26, 53, 66, 67, 68, 70, 73, 82	L	(Cervix)	100B
Human papillomavirus types 30, 34, 69, 85, 97	L		100B
Human papillomavirus, genus-beta types(except 5 and 8) and gamma types	I	(Skin)	90, 100B
Human papillomavirus types 5, 8 (in patients with epidermodysplasia verruciformis)	L	(Skin)	100B
Human immunodeficiency virus 1	S	Anus, Kaposi's sarcoma, cervix, eye, leukemia/ lymphoma, (liver/bile duct), (skin), (vulva), (vagina), (penis)	67, 100B
Human immunodeficiency virus 2	L		67
Human T-cell lymphotrophic virus I	S	Adult T-cell leukemia/ lymphoma	67, 100B
Human T-cell lymphotrophic virus II	I		67
Epstein–Barr virus	S	Nasopharynx, leukemia/ lymphoma, (stomach)	70, 100B
Human herpes virus 8	S	(Kaposi's sarcoma), leukemia/lymphoma	70, 100B
Merkel cell polyomavirus	L	(Skin)	104

(continued)

Table 5.1 (continued)

	Evidence[a]	Target organs[b]	IARC Monographs volume
Bacterium			
Helicobacter pylori	S	Stomach, leukemia/ lymphoma	61, 100B
Parasites			
Schistosoma haematobium	S	Bladder	61, 100B
Schistosoma japonicum	L	(Colorectum, liver/bile duct)	61
Schistosoma mansoni	I		61
Opistorchis viverrini	S	Liver/bile duct	61, 100B
Opistorchis felineus	I		61
Clonorchis sinensis	L	Liver/bile duct	61, 100B
Malaria (*Plasmodium falciparum*)	L	(Leukemia/lymphoma)	104

[a]*I* inadequate, *L* limited, *S* sufficient

[b]Established target organs without brackets; suspected target organs in brackets

such as asbestos, silica, arsenic, and polycyclic aromatic hydrocarbons (PAHs). Estimates of the global burden of cancer attributable to occupation in high-income countries result in figures in the order of 1–5 % (Doll and Peto 2005; Schottenfeld et al. 2013). In the past, almost 50 % of these were due to asbestos alone, while in recent years the impact of asbestos on lung cancer (but not yet mesothelioma) is levelling off (La Vecchia and Boffetta 2012). However, these cancers concentrate in some sectors of the population (mainly male blue-collar workers), among whom they may represent a sizable proportion of total cancers. Furthermore, unlike life-style factors, exposure is involuntary. In fact, reduction of exposure to occupational and environmental carcinogens has taken place in high-income, but also in several middle income, countries during recent decades. Still, further efforts should be made to further control exposure, particularly in low- and medium-income countries.

The available evidence suggests, in most populations, a small role of air, water, and soil pollutants. Global estimates are in the order of 1 % or less of total cancers (Doll and Peto 2005; Schottenfeld et al. 2013). This is in striking contrast with public perception, which often identifies pollution as a major cause of human cancer. However, in selected areas (e.g., residence near asbestos processing plants or in areas with drinking water contaminated by arsenic), environmental exposure to carcinogens may represent an important cancer hazard.

5.7 Reproductive Factors and Exogenous Hormones

There is a strong association between reproductive history and risk of cancer of the breast, ovary and endometrium. However, the role played by specific hormones and the mechanisms by which they act are still unclear. The reproductive factors with

Table 5.2 Occupational agents, classified by the IARC Monographs programme as carcinogenic to humans (monographs.iarc.fr)

Agents, mixture, circumstance	Main industry, use
Agents, groups of agents	
4-Aminobiphenyl	Pigment
Arsenic and arsenic compounds	Glass, metal, pesticide
Asbestos	Insulation, filter, textile
Benzene	Chemical, solvent
Benzidine	Pigment
Benzo[a]pyrene	Combustion processes
Beryllium and beryllium compounds	Aerospace
Bis(chloromethyl)ether and chloromethyl methyl ether	Chemical intermediate
1,3 Butadiene	Chemical
Cadmium and cadmium compounds	Dye/pigment
Chromium[VI] compounds	Metal plating, dye/pigment
Ethylene oxide	Sterilant
Formaldehyde	Chemical
Gallium arsenide	Microelectronics
2-Naphthylamine	Pigment
Nickel compounds	Metallurgy, alloy, catalyst
Polychlorinated biphenyls	Chemical
Radon-222 and its decay products	Mining
Silica, crystalline	Stone cutting, mining, glass, paper
Talc containing asbestiform fibres	Paper, paints
2,3,7,8 Tetrachlorodibenzo-para-dioxin	Chemical
Trichloroethylene	Solvent
Vinyl chloride	Plastics
X- and γ-radiation	Medical
Mixtures	
Coal-tar pitches	Construction, electrode
Coal-tars	Fuel
Diesel engine exhaust	Transport
Mineral oils, untreated and mildly treated	Metal
Shale oils	Shale oil production
Soots	Pigment
Wood dust	Wood
Exposure circumstances	
Aluminium production	
Manufacture of Auramine	
Boot and shoe manufacture and repair	
Chimney sweeping	
Coal gasification	
Coal-tar distillation	
Coke production	
Furniture and cabinet making	
Haematite mining (underground) with exposure to radon	
Iron and steel founding	
Isopropyl alcohol manufacture (strong-acid process)	
Manufacture of Magenta	
Painter (occupational exposure as a)	
Paving and roofing with coal-tar pitch	
Rubber industry	
Strong-inorganic-acid mists containing sulfuric acid (occupational exposure to)	

the strongest effect on breast cancer risk are parity not age at first full-term pregnancy. Nulliparity or low parity is also related to increased risk of endometrial and ovarian cancer. In contrast, high parity is associated to an increased risk of cervical cancer. Estrogenic stimulation is probably a major cause of breast cancer, as shown by the strong reduction in breast cancer risk among women enrolled in randomized trials of tamoxifen, and antiestrogenic drug. Exogenous estrogens and progestins given in combination as HRT and in steroid contraceptives increase the risk of breast and ovarian cancer (IARC 2007b). The risk is present, but considerably smaller, for use of estrogen-only HRT. In contrast, unopposed estrogens are strongly related to endometrial cancer. OC exert a consistent and long-term protection against ovarian and endometrial cancer, but current used of OC is associated to an increased risk of breast, cervical and breast cancer (IARC 2007b). Current OC use has also been associated with an excess risk of benign liver cancer and a modest increase of liver cancer (Cibula et al. 2010). No detailed estimates are available of the contribution of reproductive factors to the global burden of cancer, and given the uncertainties in the definition of the relevant circumstances of exposure, proposed figures for high-resource countries range from 3 % (Harvard Center for Cancer Prevention 1996) to 15 % (Doll and Peto 2005).

An effect of sex hormones on testicular and prostate cancer is plausible, but the epidemiological evidence is currently inadequate to draw any conclusion.

5.8 Perinatal and Growth Factors

Excess energy intake early in life is probably associated with an increased risk breast and colon cancer (Trichopoulos 1990). The role of attained height, growth factors, and other factors such as insulin resistance in this association is unclear. In addition, high birth weight is possibly associated with an increased risk of breast, prostate cancer and head and neck cancer. The implications of these findings for preventive strategies will be clarified by a more complete understanding of the underlying carcinogenic mechanisms.

5.9 Ionizing and Non-ionizing Radiation

Ionizing radiation causes several neoplasms, including in particular acute lymphocytic leukaemia, acute and chronic myeloid leukaemia and cancers of the breast, lung, bone, brain and thyroid (IARC 2000). Theoretical considerations and extrapolations from high doses lead to the conclusion that is a threshold below which no excess cancer risk is present is unlikely, although the quantification of the excess risk at low doses, at which most people are commonly exposed, is difficult. For most individuals, the main exposure is natural radiation, including indoor radon, although artificial sources (e.g., radiotherapy) might be important in particular cases. The estimates of the contribution of ionizing radiation to human cancer in high-resource countries are in the order of 3 % (Harvard Center for Cancer Prevention 1996) to 5 % (Doll and Peto 2005).

Solar (ultraviolet, UV) radiation is carcinogenic to the skin. Over 90 % of skin neoplasms are attributable to sunlight; because of the low fatality of non-melanocytic skin cancer, solar radiation is responsible for only about 1 % of total cancer deaths (Doll and Peto 2005). Avoidance of sun exposure, in particular during childhood, is an important cancer preventive behaviour. The evidence of a carcinogenic effect of other types of non-ionizing radiation, in particular electric and magnetic fields, is inconclusive and ionizing likely negligible, if any (Chang et al. 2014).

5.10 Medical Procedures and Drugs

The drugs that may cause or prevent cancer fall into several groups. Many cancer chemotherapy drugs are active on the DNA, which might also result in damage to normal cells. The main neoplasm associated with chemotherapy treatment is leukaemia, although the risk of solid tumours might also be increased. A second group of carcinogenic drugs includes immunosuppressive agents, notably used in transplanted patients. NHL is the main neoplasm caused by these drugs. The carcinogenic effects of HRT and OC are discussed above. Phenacetin-containing analgesics increase the risk of cancer of the renal pelvis.

No precise estimates are available for the global contribution of drug use to human cancer. It is unlikely, however, that they represent more than 1 % in high-resource countries (Doll and Peto 2005). Furthermore, the benefits of therapies are usually much greater than the potential cancer risk.

Use of ionizing radiation for diagnostic purposes is likely to carry a small risk of cancer, which has been demonstrated only for childhood leukaemia following intrauterine exposure. Radiotherapy increases the risk of cancer in the irradiated organs. There is no evidence of an increased cancer risk following other medical procedures, including mammography and surgical implants.

Chemoprevention can also be considered for primary and secondary prevention of cancer, but data are negative or inconsistent for most micronutrients or other substances considered.

Data are however more promising for aspirin. In fact, aspirin has been associated to a reduced risk of colorectal and possibly of a few other common cancers, but quantification remains open to discussion (Cuzick et al. 2009). A meta-analysis of observational studies on aspirin and 12 cancer sites published up to September 2011 included a total of 139 studies (Bosetti et al. 2012d). Regular aspirin is associated with a reduced risk of colorectal cancer [summary relative risk (RR) based on over 30,000 cases = 0.73, 95 % confidence interval (CI) 0.67–0.79], and of other digestive tract cancers (RR = 0.61, 95 % CI = 0.50–0.76, for squamous cell esophageal cancer; RR = 0.64, 95 % CI = 0.52–0.78, for esophageal and gastric cardia adenocarcinoma; and RR = 0.67, 95 % CI = 0.54–0.83, for gastric cancer). Modest inverse associations were also observed for breast (RR=0.90, 95 % CI=0.85–0.95) and prostate cancer (RR=0.90, 95 % CI=0.85–0.96), while lung cancer was significantly reduced in case–control studies (0.73, 95 % CI=0.55–0.98) but not in cohort ones (RR=0.98, 95 % CI=0.92–1.05). No meaningful associations were observed for cancers of the pancreas, endometrium, ovary, bladder, and kidney. Thus, a large number of observational studies, but also evidence from prospective clinical trials (Rothwell et al. 2011) indicate a beneficial role of aspirin on colorectal and other digestive tract cancers; modest risk reductions were also observed for breast and prostate cancer.

5.11 Genetic Factors

A number of inherited mutations of a high-penetrance cancer gene increase dramatically the risk of some neoplasms. However, these are rare conditions in most populations and the number of cases attributable to them is rather small.

Familial aggregation has been shown for most types of cancers, in non-carriers of known high-penetrance genes. This is notably the case for cancers of the breast, colon, prostate and lung. The RR is in the order of 2–4, and is higher for cases diagnosed at young age. Although some of the aggregation can be explained by shared risk factors among family members, it is plausible that a true genetic component exists for most human cancers. This takes the forms of an increased susceptibility to endogenous and exogenous carcinogens. The effect on cancer risk of common genetic variants with a small to moderate risk of cancer (approximately twofold) responsible for such susceptibility has been extensively studied in the past two decades within genetic association studies. Some synopsis have been published mostly regarding genes involved in the DNA repair, encoding for metabolic enzymes and cell cycle control (Vineis et al. 2009). Despite many years of candidate gene studies testing for gene–environment interaction, however, there are only few notable replicated and widely-agreed-upon examples of success (e.g., NAT2, smoking, and bladder cancer; ALDH2, alcohol and esophageal cancer), as publication bias and false positive findings largely affected the literature in this field.

In recent years, with the advent of Genome Wide Association Studies (GWAS) that use an agnostic approach identified new genes that might confer cancer susceptibility, though their clinical utility is currently very limited (Stadler et al. 2010).

Chapter 6
Conclusions

Keywords Cancer prevention • Cancer control

Neoplasms are a group of diverse diseases with complex distributions in human populations and with different aetiological factors. Current knowledge of the causes of human neoplasms and the development of control strategies have led to the elaboration of lists of recommendations for their prevention (Table 6.1). A comprehensive strategy for cancer control might lead to the avoidance of a sizeable proportion of human cancers, and the greatest benefit can be achieved via tobacco control. However, such a strategy would imply major cultural, societal and economic changes. More modest objectives for cancer prevention should focus on the neoplasms and the exposures that are prevalent in any given population. For example, vaccination of children against HBV and adolescents woman against HPV are likely to be the most cost-effective cancer prevention action in many countries of Africa and Asia.

Neoplasms will continue to be a major source of human disease and death. Considerable efforts are made in the public and private domains to develop effective therapeutic approaches for a wide number of important neoplasms. Even if major discoveries in the clinical management of cancer patients will be accomplished in the near future, the changes will mainly affect the affluent part of the world population. Prevention of the known causes of cancer remains the most promising approach in reducing the consequences of cancer, in particular in countries with limited resources. Control of tobacco smoking and of smokeless tobacco products, reduced overweight and obesity, moderation in alcohol intake, increased physical activity, avoidance of exposure to solar radiation in central hours of the days in summer and control of known occupational (Chang et al. 2014) carcinogens are the main approaches, we currently have to reduce the burden of human neoplasms.

P. Boffetta et al., *A Quick Guide to Cancer Epidemiology*, SpringerBriefs in Cancer Research, DOI 10.1007/978-3-319-05068-3_6,

Table 6.1 European Code Against Cancer (Boyle et al. 2003)

Many aspects of general health can be improved, and many cancer deaths prevented, if we adopt healthier lifestyles:

1. Do not smoke; if you smoke, stop doing so. If you fail to stop, do not smoke in the presence of non-smokers.
2. Avoid obesity.
3. Undertake some brisk, physical activity every day.
4. Increase your daily intake and variety of vegetables and fruits: eat at least five servings daily. Limit your intake of foods containing fats from animal sources.
5. If you drink alcohol, whether beer, wine or spirits, moderate your consumption to two drinks per day if you are a man or one drink per day if you are a woman.
6. Care must be taken to avoid excessive sun exposure. It is specifically important to protect children and adolescents. For individuals who have a tendency to burn in the sun active protective measures must be taken throughout life.
7. Apply strictly regulations aimed at preventing any exposure to known cancer-causing substances. Follow all health and safety instructions on substances which may cause cancer. Follow advice of National Radiation Protection Offices.

There are public health programmes that could prevent cancers developing or increase the probability that a cancer may be cured:

8. Women from 25 years of age should participate in cervical screening. This should be within programmes with quality control procedures in compliance with *European Guidelines for Quality Assurance in Cervical Screening*.
9. Women from 50 years of age should participate in breast screening. This should be within programmes with quality control procedures in compliance with *European Guidelines for Quality Assurance in Mammography Screening*.
10. Men and women from 50 years of age should participate in colorectal screening. This should be within programmes with built-in quality assurance procedures.
11. Participate in vaccination programmes against hepatitis B virus infection.

References

Aberle DR, Adams AM, Berg CD, Black WC, Clapp JD, Fagerstrom RM et al (2011) Reduced lung-cancer mortality with low-dose computed tomographic screening. N Engl J Med 365: 395–409

Adami HO, Hunter DJ, Trichopoulous D (2008) Textbook of cancer epidemiology, 2nd edn. Oxford University Press, New York

Albanes D, Heinonen OP, Taylor PR, Virtamo J, Edwards BK, Rautalahti M et al (1996) Alpha-Tocopherol and beta-carotene supplements and lung cancer incidence in the alpha-tocopherol, beta-carotene cancer prevention study: effects of base-line characteristics and study compliance. J Natl Cancer Inst 88:1560–1570

Alexander DD, Morimoto LM, Mink PJ, Lowe KA (2010) Summary and meta-analysis of prospective studies of animal fat intake and breast cancer. Nutr Res Rev 23:169–179

Altieri A, Franceschi S, Ferlay J, Smith J, La Vecchia C (2003) Epidemiology and aetiology of gestational trophoblastic diseases. Lancet Oncol 4:670–678

Amundadottir LT, Sulem P, Gudmundsson J, Helgason A, Baker A, Agnarsson BA et al (2006) A common variant associated with prostate cancer in European and African populations. Nat Genet 38:652–658

Anderson K, Mack T, Silverman D (2006) Cancer of the pancreas. In: Schottenfeld D, Fraumeni JF (eds) Cancer epidemiology and prevention. Oxford University Press, New York, pp 721–762

Anttila A, Sarkeala T, Hakulinen T, Heinavaara S (2008) Impacts of the Finnish service screening programme on breast cancer rates. BMC Public Health 8:38

Appleby P, Beral V, Berrington de Gonzalez A, Colin D, Franceschi S, Goodhill A et al (2007) Cervical cancer and hormonal contraceptives: collaborative reanalysis of individual data for 16,573 women with cervical cancer and 35,509 women without cervical cancer from 24 epidemiological studies. Lancet 370:1609–1621

Armstrong BK, Kricker A (2007) Sun exposure and non-Hodgkin lymphoma. Cancer Epidemiol Biomarkers Prev 16:396–400

Assi V, Warwick J, Cuzick J, Duffy SW (2012) Clinical and epidemiological issues in mammographic density. Nat Rev Clin Oncol 9:33–40

Aune D, Lau R, Chan DS, Vieira R, Greenwood DC, Kampman E et al (2012) Dairy products and colorectal cancer risk: a systematic review and meta-analysis of cohort studies. Ann Oncol 23:37–45

Baan R, Straif K, Grosse Y, Secretan B, El Ghissassi F, Bouvard V et al (2007) Carcinogenicity of alcoholic beverages. Lancet Oncol 8:292–293

Bagnardi V, Rota M, Botteri E, Tramacere I, Islami F, Fedirko V et al (2013) Light alcohol drinking and cancer: a meta-analysis. Ann Oncol 24:301–308

P. Boffetta et al., *A Quick Guide to Cancer Epidemiology*, SpringerBriefs in Cancer Research, DOI 10.1007/978-3-319-05068-3,

Baili P, Micheli A, De Angelis R, Weir HK, Francisci S, Santaquilani M et al (2008) Life tables for world-wide comparison of relative survival for cancer (CONCORD study). Tumori 94: 658–668

Bedwani R, Renganathan E, El Kwhsky F, Braga C, Abu Seif HH, Abul Azm T et al (1998) Schistosomiasis and the risk of bladder cancer in Alexandria, Egypt. Br J Cancer 77: 1186–1189

Beebe-Dimer J, Schottenfeld D (2006) Cancers of the small intestine. In: Schottenfeld D, Fraumeni JF (eds) Cancer epidemiology and prevention. Oxford University Press, New York, pp 801–808

Bergstrom A, Pisani P, Tenet V, Wolk A, Adami HO (2001) Overweight as an avoidable cause of cancer in Europe. Int J Cancer 91:421–430

Bertuccio P, Malvezzi M, Chatenoud L, Bosetti C, Negri E, Levi F et al (2007) Testicular cancer mortality in the Americas, 1980–2003. Cancer 109:776–779

Bertuccio P, La Vecchia C, Silverman DT, Petersen GM, Bracci PM, Negri E et al (2011) Cigar and pipe smoking, smokeless tobacco use and pancreatic cancer: an analysis from the International Pancreatic Cancer Case-Control Consortium (PanC4). Ann Oncol 22:1420–1426

Berwick M (2006) Soft tissue sarcoma. In: Schottenfeld D, Fraumeni JF (eds) Cancer epidemiology and prevention. Oxford University Press, New York, pp 959–974

Blot WJ (1997) Vitamin/mineral supplementation and cancer risk: international chemoprevention trials. Proc Soc Exp Biol Med 216:291–296

Blot W, McLaughlin J, Fraumeni J (2006) Esophageal cancer. In: Schottenfeld D, Fraumeni JF (eds) Cancer epidemiology and prevention. Oxford University Press, New York, pp 697–706

Boccia S, La Vecchia C (2013) Dissecting causal components in gastric carcinogenesis. Eur J Cancer Prev 22:489–491

Boccia S, La Torre G, Gianfagna F, Mannocci A, Ricciardi G (2006) Glutathione S-transferase T1 status and gastric cancer risk: a meta-analysis of the literature. Mutagenesis 21:115–123

Boffetta P (2006) Human cancer from environmental pollutants: the epidemiological evidence. Mutat Res 608:157–162

Boffetta P, Hashibe M (2006) Alcohol and cancer. Lancet Oncol 7:149–156

Boffetta P, Islami F (2013) The contribution of molecular epidemiology to the identification of human carcinogens: current status and future perspectives. Ann Oncol 24:901–908

Boffetta P, La Vecchia C (2009) Neoplasms. In: Detels R, Beaglehole R, Lansang MA, Gulliford M (eds) The practice of public health. Oxford textbook of public health, 5th edn, vol 3. Oxford University Press, New York, pp 997–1020

Boffetta P, Stayner L (2006) Pleural and peritoneal neoplasms. In: Schottenfeld D, Fraumeni JF (eds) Cancer epidemiology and prevention. Oxford University Press, New York, pp 659–673

Boffetta P, Hecht S, Gray N, Gupta P, Straif K (2008) Smokeless tobacco and cancer. Lancet Oncol 9:667–675

Bosetti C, Kolonel L, Negri E, Ron E, Franceschi S, Dal Maso L et al (2001) A pooled analysis of case-control studies of thyroid cancer. VI. Fish and shellfish consumption. Cancer Causes Control 12:375–382

Bosetti C, Negri E, Kolonel L, Ron E, Franceschi S, Preston-Martin S et al (2002) A pooled analysis of case-control studies of thyroid cancer. VII. Cruciferous and other vegetables (International). Cancer Causes Control 13:765–775

Bosetti C, Malvezzi M, Chatenoud L, Negri E, Levi F, La Vecchia C (2005) Trends in cancer mortality in the Americas, 1970–2000. Ann Oncol 16:489–511

Bosetti C, Gallus S, Garavello W, La Vecchia C (2006) Smoking cessation and the risk of oesophageal cancer: an overview of published studies. Oral Oncol 42:957–964

Bosetti C, Gallus S, Peto R, Negri E, Talamini R, Tavani A et al (2008a) Tobacco smoking, smoking cessation, and cumulative risk of upper aerodigestive tract cancers. Am J Epidemiol 167:468–473

Bosetti C, Levi F, Ferlay J, Garavello W, Lucchini F, Bertuccio P et al (2008b) Trends in oesophageal cancer incidence and mortality in Europe. Int J Cancer 122:1118–1129

Bosetti C, Bertuccio P, Chatenoud L, Negri E, La Vecchia C, Levi F (2011) Trends in mortality from urologic cancers in Europe, 1970–2008. Eur Urol 60:1–15

Bosetti C, Bertuccio P, Negri E, La Vecchia C, Zeegers MP, Boffetta P (2012a) Pancreatic cancer: overview of descriptive epidemiology. Mol Carcinog 51:3–13

Bosetti C, Lucenteforte E, Silverman DT, Petersen G, Bracci PM, Ji BT et al (2012b) Cigarette smoking and pancreatic cancer: an analysis from the International Pancreatic Cancer Case-Control Consortium (Panc4). Ann Oncol 23:1880–1888

Bosetti C, Malvezzi M, Rosso T, Bertuccio P, Gallus S, Chatenoud L et al (2012c) Lung cancer mortality in European women: trends and predictions. Lung Cancer 78:171–178

Bosetti C, Rosato V, Gallus S, Cuzick J, La Vecchia C (2012d) Aspirin and cancer risk: a quantitative review to 2011. Ann Oncol 23:1403–1415

Bosetti C, Bertuccio P, Malvezzi M, Levi F, Chatenoud L, Negri E et al (2013) Cancer mortality in Europe, 2005–2009, and an overview of trends since 1980. Ann Oncol 24:2657–2671

Boyle P, Brawley OW (2009) Prostate cancer: current evidence weighs against population screening. CA Cancer J Clin 59:220–224

Boyle P, Autier P, Bartelink H, Baselga J, Boffetta P, Burn J et al (2003) European Code Against Cancer and scientific justification: third version (2003). Ann Oncol 14:973–1005

Bravi F, Edefonti V, Randi G, Garavello W, La Vecchia C, Ferraroni M et al (2012) Dietary patterns and the risk of esophageal cancer. Ann Oncol 23:765–770

Burningham Z, Hashibe M, Spector L, Schiffman JD (2012) The epidemiology of sarcoma. Clin Sarcoma Res 2:14

Chan AT, Giovannucci EL (2010) Primary prevention of colorectal cancer. Gastroenterology 138:2029–2043.e2010

Chan DS, Lau R, Aune D, Vieira R, Greenwood DC, Kampman E et al (2011) Red and processed meat and colorectal cancer incidence: meta-analysis of prospective studies. PLoS One 6:e20456

Chang E, Adami HO, Bailey WH, Boffetta P, Krieger RI, Moolgavkar SH et al (2014) Validity of geographically modeled environmental exposure estimates. Critical Rev Toxicol

Chatenoud L, Bertuccio P, Bosetti C, Levi F, Negri E, La Vecchia C (2010) Childhood cancer mortality in America, Asia, and Oceania, 1970 through 2007. Cancer 116:5063–5074

Chatenoud L, Bertuccio P, Bosetti C, Rodriguez T, Levi F, Negri E et al (2013) Hodgkin's lymphoma mortality in the Americas, 1997–2008: achievements and persistent inadequacies. Int J Cancer. doi:10.1002/ijc.28049

Chen GC, Pang Z, Liu QF (2012) Magnesium intake and risk of colorectal cancer: a meta-analysis of prospective studies. Eur J Clin Nutr 66:1182–1186

Chlebowski RT, Hendrix SL, Langer RD, Stefanick ML, Gass M, Lane D et al (2003) Influence of estrogen plus progestin on breast cancer and mammography in healthy postmenopausal women: the Women's Health Initiative Randomized Trial. JAMA 289:3243–3253

Cibula D, Gompel A, Mueck AO, La Vecchia C, Hannaford PC, Skouby SO et al (2010) Hormonal contraception and risk of cancer. Hum Reprod Update 16:631–650

Clifford GM, Gallus S, Herrero R, Munoz N, Snijders PJ, Vaccarella S et al (2005) Worldwide distribution of human papillomavirus types in cytologically normal women in the International Agency for Research on Cancer HPV prevalence surveys: a pooled analysis. Lancet 366: 991–998

Colditz G, Baer H, Tamimi R (2006) Breast cancer. In: Schottenfeld D, Fraumeni JF (eds) Cancer epidemiology and prevention. Oxford University Press, New York, pp 995–1012

Collaborative Group on Epidemiological Studies of Ovarian Cancer (2012) Ovarian cancer and body size: individual participant meta-analysis including 25,157 women with ovarian cancer from 47 epidemiological studies. PLoS Med 9:e1001200

Collaborative Group on Epidemiological Studies of Ovarian Cancer, Beral V, Doll R, Hermon C, Peto R, Reeves G (2008) Ovarian cancer and oral contraceptives: collaborative reanalysis of data from 45 epidemiological studies including 23,257 women with ovarian cancer and 87,303 controls. Lancet 371:303–314

Collaborative Group on Epidemiological Studies of Ovarian Cancer, Beral V, Gaitskell K, Hermon C, Moser K, Reeves G et al (2012) Ovarian cancer and smoking: individual participant meta-analysis including 28,114 women with ovarian cancer from 51 epidemiological studies. Lancet Oncol 13:946–956

Collaborative Group on Hormonal Factors Breast Cancer (2002) Breast cancer and breastfeeding: collaborative reanalysis of individual data from 47 epidemiological studies in 30 countries, including 50302 women with breast cancer and 96973 women without the disease. Lancet 360:187–195

Conway DI, Petticrew M, Marlborough H, Berthiller J, Hashibe M, Macpherson LM (2008) Socioeconomic inequalities and oral cancer risk: a systematic review and meta-analysis of case-control studies. Int J Cancer 122:2811–2819

Cook L, Weis NS, Doherty JA, Chen C (2006) Endometrial cancer. In: Schottenfeld D, Fraumeni JF (eds) Cancer epidemiology and prevention. Oxford University Press, New York, pp 1027–1043

Cuzick J (2010) Long-term cervical cancer prevention strategies across the globe. Gynecol Oncol 117:S11–S14

Cuzick J, Otto F, Baron JA, Brown PH, Burn J, Greenwald P et al (2009) Aspirin and non-steroidal anti-inflammatory drugs for cancer prevention: an international consensus statement. Lancet Oncol 10:501–507

Dal Maso L, Bosetti C, La Vecchia C, Franceschi S (2009) Risk factors for thyroid cancer: an epidemiological review focused on nutritional factors. Cancer Causes Control 20:75–86

Darby S, Hill D, Auvinen A, Barros-Dios JM, Baysson H, Bochicçhio F et al (2005) Radon in homes and risk of lung cancer: collaborative analysis of individual data from 13 European case–control studies. BMJ 330:223

de Martel C, Ferlay J, Franceschi S, Vignat J, Bray F, Forman D et al (2012) Global burden of cancers attributable to infections in 2008: a review and synthetic analysis. Lancet Oncol 13:607–615

Doll R, Peto R (2005) Epidemiology of cancer. In: Warell DA, Cox TM, Firth JD (eds) Oxford textbook of medicine, vol 3, 4th edn. Oxford University Press, New York, pp 193–218

Doll R, Peto R, Boreham J, Sutherland I (2004) Mortality in relation to smoking: 50 years' observations on male British doctors. BMJ 328:1519

El-Serag HB (2004) Hepatocellular carcinoma: recent trends in the United States. Gastroenterology 127:S27–S34

Ferlay J, Bray F, Pisani P, Parkin DM (2004) GLOBOCAN 2002. Cancer incidence, mortality and prevalence worldwide IARC Cancer Base No. 5 [Internet]. Version 2.0. IARC, Lyon

Ferlay J, Shin HR, Bray F, Forman D, Mathers C, Parkin DM (2010a) Estimates of worldwide burden of cancer in 2008: GLOBOCAN 2008. Int J Cancer 127:2893–2917

Ferlay J, Shin HR, Bray F, Forman D, Mathers C, Parkin DM (2010b) GLOBOCAN 2008 v2.0. Cancer incidence and mortality worldwide: IARC Cancer Base No.10 [Internet]. International Agency for Research on Cancer, Lyon

Ferlay J, Soerjomataram I, Ervik M, Dikshit R, Eser S, Mathers C, Rebelo M, Parkin DM, Forman D, Bray F (2013) GLOBOCAN 2012 v1.0. Cancer incidence and mortality worldwide: IARC Cancer Base No. 11 [Internet]. International Agency for Research on Cancer, Lyon

Fernandez E, La Vecchia C, Gonzalez JR, Lucchini F, Negri E, Levi F (2005) Converging patterns of colorectal cancer mortality in Europe. Eur J Cancer 41:430–437

Forman D, Bray F, Brewster DH, Gombe Mbalawa C, Kohler B, Piñeros M, Steliarova-Foucher E, Swaminathan R, Ferlay J (eds) (2013) Cancer incidence in five continents, vol X (electronic version). IARC, Lyon

Franceschi S, Preston-Martin S, Dal Maso L, Negri E, La Vecchia C, Mack WJ et al (1999) A pooled analysis of case-control studies of thyroid cancer. IV. Benign thyroid diseases. Cancer Causes Control 10:583–595

Frisch M, Melbye M (2006) Anal cancer. In: Schottenfeld D, Fraumeni JF (eds) Cancer epidemiology and prevention. Oxford University Press, New York, pp 830–840

FUTURE II Study Group (2007) Quadrivalent vaccine against human papillomavirus to prevent high-grade cervical lesions. N Engl J Med 356:1915–1927

Galeone C, Malerba S, Rota M, Bagnardi V, Negri E, Scotti L et al (2013) A meta-analysis of alcohol consumption and the risk of brain tumours. Ann Oncol 24:514–523

Gandini S, Botteri E, Iodice S, Boniol M, Lowenfels AB, Maisonneuve P et al (2008) Tobacco smoking and cancer: a meta-analysis. Int J Cancer 122:155–164

Garavello W, Negri E, Talamini R, Levi F, Zambon P, Dal Maso L et al (2005) Family history of cancer, its combination with smoking and drinking, and risk of squamous cell carcinoma of the esophagus. Cancer Epidemiol Biomarkers Prev 14:1390–1393

Garcia-Closas M, Malats N, Silverman D, Dosemeci M, Kogevinas M, Hein DW et al (2005) NAT2 slow acetylation, GSTM1 null genotype, and risk of bladder cancer: results from the Spanish Bladder Cancer Study and meta-analyses. Lancet 366:649–659

Garcia-Closas M, Rothman N, Figueroa JD, Prokunina-Olsson L, Han SS, Baris D et al (2013) Common genetic polymorphisms modify the effect of smoking on absolute risk of bladder cancer. Cancer Res 73:2211–2220

Gauderman WJ, Morrison JL, Carpenter CL, Thomas DC (1997) Analysis of gene-smoking interaction in lung cancer. Genet Epidemiol 14:199–214

Giovannucci E (2005) The epidemiology of vitamin D and cancer incidence and mortality: a review (United States). Cancer Causes Control 16:83–95

Gokmen MR, Cosyns JP, Arlt VM, Stiborova M, Phillips DH, Schmeiser HH et al (2013) The epidemiology, diagnosis, and management of aristolochic acid nephropathy: a narrative review. Ann Intern Med 158:469–477

Greenwald P (2005) Lifestyle and medical approaches to cancer prevention. Recent Results Cancer Res 166:1–15

Grodstein F, Speizer FE, Hunter DJ (1995) A prospective study of incident squamous cell carcinoma of the skin in the nurses' health study. J Natl Cancer Inst 87:1061–1066

Gruber S, Armstrong B (2006) Cutaneous and ocular melanoma. In: Schottenfeld D, Fraumeni JF (eds) Cancer epidemiology and prevention. Oxford University Press, New York, pp 1196–1229

Gudmundsson J, Sulem P, Manolescu A, Amundadottir LT, Gudbjartsson D, Helgason A et al (2007a) Genome-wide association study identifies a second prostate cancer susceptibility variant at 8q24. Nat Genet 39:631–637

Gudmundsson J, Sulem P, Steinthorsdottir V, Bergthorsson JT, Thorleifsson G, Manolescu A et al (2007b) Two variants on chromosome 17 confer prostate cancer risk, and the one in TCF2 protects against type 2 diabetes. Nat Genet 39:977–983

Haiman CA, Patterson N, Freedman ML, Myers SR, Pike MC, Waliszewska A et al (2007) Multiple regions within 8q24 independently affect risk for prostate cancer. Nat Genet 39: 638–644

Hanahan D, Weinberg RA (2011) Hallmarks of cancer: the next generation. Cell 144:646–674

Hankinson S, Danforth K (2006) Ovarian. In: Schottenfeld D, Fraumeni JF (eds) Cancer epidemiology and prevention. Oxford University Press, New York, pp 1013–1026

Hartge P, Wang S, Bracci M, Devesa S, Holly E (2006) Non Hodgkin lymphoma. In: Schottenfeld D, Fraumeni JF (eds) Cancer epidemiology and prevention. Oxford University Press, New York, pp 898–918

Harvard Center for Cancer Prevention (1996) Harvard report on cancer prevention. Volume 1: causes of human cancer. Cancer Causes Control 7(suppl 1):S3–59

Hemminki K, Hussain S (2008) Mesothelioma incidence has leveled off in Sweden. Int J Cancer 122:1200–1201

Hsing AW, Rashid A, Devesa SS, Fraumeni JF (2006) Biliary tract cancer. In: Schottenfeld D, Fraumeni JF (eds) Cancer epidemiology and prevention. Oxford University Press, New York, pp 787–800

Hystad P, Demers PA, Johnson KC, Carpiano RM, Brauer M (2013) Long-term residential exposure to air pollution and lung cancer risk. Epidemiology 24:762–772

IARC (1996) Human immunodeficiency viruses. In: IARC monographs on the evaluation of carcinogenic risks to humans. Human immunodeficiency viruses and human T-cell lymphotropic viruses, vol 67. IARC, Lyon, pp 31–183

IARC (1997) Epstein–Barr virus and Kaposi's sarcoma herpesvirus/human herpesvirus 8. In: Epstein–Barr virus. IARC monographs on the evaluation of carcinogenic risks to humans, vol 70. IARC, Lyon, pp 47–374

IARC (1998a) Carotenoids. In: IARC handbooks of cancer prevention, vol 2. IARC, Lyon, pp 1–326

IARC (1998b) Vitamin A. In: IARC handbooks of cancer prevention, vol 3. IARC, Lyon, pp 1–261

IARC (2000) X-radiation and y-radiation. In: IARC monographs on the evaluation of carcinogenic risks to humans. Ionizing radiation, part 1: X- and Gamma (y)-radiation, and neutrons, vol 75. IARC, Lyon, pp 121–362

IARC (2001) Ionizing radiation, part 2: some internally deposited radionuclides. In: IARC monographs on the evaluation of carcinogenic risks to humans, vol 78. IARC, Lyon, pp 1–563

IARC (2002) Weight control and physical activity. In: IARC handbooks of cancer prevention, vol 6. IARC, Lyon, pp 1–315

IARC (2004) Tobacco smoke and involuntary smoking. In: IARC monographs on the evaluation of the carcinogenic risks to humans, vol 83. IARC, Lyon, pp 51–1187

IARC (2007a) In: Curado MP, Shin HR, Storm H, Ferlay J, Heanue M, Boyle P (eds). Cancer incidence in five continents, vol. IX. International Agency for Research on Cancer, Lyon

IARC (2007b) Combined estrogen-progestogen contraceptives and combined estrogen-progestogen menopausal therapy. In: IARC monographs on the evaluation of carcinogenic risks to humans, vol 91. IARC, Lyon

IARC (2008) In: Vitamin D and cancer/a report of the IARC working group on vitamin D, vol 5. IARC, Lyon

IARC (2010) Household combustion of solid fuels and high-temperature frying. In: IARC monographs on the evaluation of carcinogenic risks to humans, vol 95. IARC, Lyon

Islami F, Fedirko V, Tramacere I, Bagnardi V, Jenab M, Scotti L et al (2011) Alcohol drinking and esophageal squamous cell carcinoma with focus on light-drinkers and never-smokers: a systematic review and meta-analysis. Int J Cancer 129:2473–2484

IUKPBCS (2012) The benefits and harms of breast cancer screening: an independent review. Lancet 380:1778–1786

Jaffe ES, Harris NL, Stein H, Isaacson PG (2008) Classification of lymphoid neoplasms: the microscope as a tool for disease discovery. Blood 112:4384–4399

Jepsen P, Vilstrup H, Tarone RE, Friis S, Sorensen HT (2007) Incidence rates of intra- and extrahepatic cholangiocarcinomas in Denmark from 1978 through 2002. J Natl Cancer Inst 99:895–897

Jha P, Ramasundarahettige C, Landsman V, Rostron B, Thun M, Anderson RN et al (2013) 21st-century hazards of smoking and benefits of cessation in the United States. N Engl J Med 368:341–350

Kalager M, Zelen M, Langmark F, Adami HO (2010) Effect of screening mammography on breast-cancer mortality in Norway. N Engl J Med 363:1203–1210

Karagas M, Weinstock M, Nelson H (2006) Keratinocyte carcinomas (basal and squamous cell carcinomas of the skin). In: Schottenfeld D, Fraumeni JF (eds) Cancer epidemiology and prevention. Oxford University Press, New York, pp 1230–1250

Kato I, Canzian F, Plummer M, Franceschi S, van Doorn LJ, Vivas J et al (2007) Polymorphisms in genes related to bacterial lipopolysaccharide/peptidoglycan signaling and gastric precancerous lesions in a population at high risk for gastric cancer. Dig Dis Sci 52:254–261

La Vecchia C (2006) Estrogen-progestogen replacement therapy and ovarian cancer: an update. Eur J Cancer Prev 15:490–492

La Vecchia C (2007) Alcohol and liver cancer. Eur J Cancer Prev 16:495–497

La Vecchia C, Boffetta P (2012) Role of stopping exposure and recent exposure to asbestos in the risk of mesothelioma. Eur J Cancer Prev 21:227–230

La Vecchia C, Bosetti C (2003) Oral contraceptives and cervical cancer: public health implications. Eur J Cancer Prev 12:1–2

La Vecchia C, Franceschi S, Decarli A, Fasoli M, Gentile A, Parazzini F et al (1986) Sexual factors, venereal diseases, and the risk of intraepithelial and invasive cervical neoplasia. Cancer 58:935–941

La Vecchia C, Negri E, Franceschi S, Gentile A (1992) Family history and the risk of stomach and colorectal cancer. Cancer 70:50–55

La Vecchia C, Altieri A, Franceschi S, Tavani A (2001) Oral contraceptives and cancer: an update. Drug Saf 24:741–754

La Vecchia C, Negri E, Lagiou P, Trichopoulos D (2002) Oesophageal adenocarcinoma: a paradigm of mechanical carcinogenesis? Int J Cancer 102:269–270

La Vecchia C, Bosetti C, Lucchini F, Bertuccio P, Negri E, Boyle P et al (2010) Cancer mortality in Europe, 2000–2004, and an overview of trends since 1975. Ann Oncol 21:1323–1360

Ladeiras-Lopes R, Pereira AK, Nogueira A, Pinheiro-Torres T, Pinto I, Santos-Pereira R et al (2008) Smoking and gastric cancer: systematic review and meta-analysis of cohort studies. Cancer Causes Control 19:689–701

Lagiou P, Adami HO, Trichopoulos D (2006) Early life diet and the risk for adult breast cancer. Nutr Cancer 56:158–161

Lee IM, Shiroma EJ, Lobelo F, Puska P, Blair SN, Katzmarzyk PT (2012) Effect of physical inactivity on major non-communicable diseases worldwide: an analysis of burden of disease and life expectancy. Lancet 380:219–229

Leoncini E, Ricciardi W, Cadoni G, Arzani D, Petrelli L, Paludetti G et al (2014) Adult height and head and neck cancer: a pooled analysis within the INHANCE Consortium. Eur J Epidemiol 29:35–48

Levi F, Te VC, Randimbison L, Erler G, La Vecchia C (2001) Trends in skin cancer incidence in Vaud: an update, 1976–1998. Eur J Cancer Prev 10:371–373

Levi F, Lucchini F, Boyle P, Negri E, La Vecchia C (2003) Testicular cancer mortality in Eastern Europe. Int J Cancer 105:574

Levi F, Lucchini F, Negri E, La Vecchia C (2004) Declining mortality from kidney cancer in Europe. Ann Oncol 15:1130–1135

Levi F, Randimbison L, Maspoli M, Te VC, La Vecchia C (2006) High incidence of second basal cell skin cancers. Int J Cancer 119:1505–1507

Lewis SJ, Smith GD (2005) Alcohol, ALDH2, and esophageal cancer: a meta-analysis which illustrates the potentials and limitations of a Mendelian randomization approach. Cancer Epidemiol Biomarkers Prev 14:1967–1971

Li H, Stampfer MJ, Hollis JB, Mucci LA, Gaziano JM, Hunter D et al (2007) A prospective study of plasma vitamin D metabolites, vitamin D receptor polymorphisms, and prostate cancer. PLoS Med 4:e103

Li X, Gao L, Li H, Gao J, Yang Y, Zhou F et al (2013) Human papillomavirus infection and laryngeal cancer risk: a systematic review and meta-analysis. J Infect Dis 207:479–488

Linet M, Devesa S, Morgan G (2007) The leukemias. In: Schottenfeld D, Fraumeni JF (eds) Cancer epidemiology and prevention. Oxford University Press, Lyon, pp 841–871

Littman A, Vaughan T (2006) Cancers of the nasal cavity and paranasal sinuses. In: Schottenfeld D, Fraumeni JF (eds) Cancer epidemiology and prevention. Oxford University Press, New York, pp 603–619

Liu L, Zhuang W, Wang RQ, Mukherjee R, Xiao SM, Chen Z et al (2011) Is dietary fat associated with the risk of colorectal cancer? A meta-analysis of 13 prospective cohort studies. Eur J Nutr 50:173–184

London W, McGlynn K (2006) Liver cancer. In: Schottenfeld D, Fraumeni JF (eds) Cancer epidemiology and prevention. Oxford University Press, New York, pp 763–786

Lubin JH, Liang Z, Hrubec Z, Pershagen G, Schoenberg JB, Blot WJ et al (1994) Radon exposure in residences and lung cancer among women: combined analysis of three studies. Cancer Causes Control 5:114–128

Madeleine M, Daling J (2006) Cancers of the vulva and vagina. In: Schottenfeld D, Fraumeni JF (eds) Cancer epidemiology and prevention. Oxford University Press, New York, pp 1068–1074

Maitra SK, Gallo H, Rowland-Payne C, Robinson D, Moller H (2005) Second primary cancers in patients with squamous cell carcinoma of the skin. Br J Cancer 92:570–571

Malvezzi M, Bertuccio P, Levi F, La Vecchia C, Negri E (2013a) European cancer mortality predictions for the year 2013. Ann Oncol 24:792–800

Malvezzi M, Bosetti C, Rosso T, Bertuccio P, Chatenoud L, Levi F et al (2013b) Lung cancer mortality in European men: trends and predictions. Lung Cancer 80:138–145

Malvezzi M, Bertuccio P, Levi F, La Vecchia C, Negri E (2014) European cancer mortality predictions for the year 2014. Ann Oncol in press

Mayne S, Morse D, Winn D (2006) Cancers of the oral cavity and pharynx. In: Schottenfeld D, Fraumeni JF (eds) Cancer epidemiology and prevention. Oxford University Press, New York, pp 674–696

McKay JD, Truong T, Gaborieau V, Chabrier A, Chuang SC, Byrnes G et al (2011) A genome-wide association study of upper aerodigestive tract cancers conducted within the INHANCE consortium. PLoS Genet 7:e1001333

McLaughlin J, Lipworth L, Tarone R, Blot W (2006) Renal cancer. In: Schottenfeld D, Fraumeni JF (eds) Cancer epidemiology and prevention. Oxford University Press, New York, pp 1087–1100

Mendez D, Alshanqeety O, Warner KE (2013) The potential impact of smoking control policies on future global smoking trends. Tob Control 22:46–51

Millen AE, Tucker MA, Hartge P, Halpern A, Elder DE, Guerry D et al (2004) Diet and melanoma in a case-control study. Cancer Epidemiol Biomarkers Prev 13:1042–1051

Miller R, Boice J, Curtis R (2006) Bone cancer. In: Schottenfeld D, Fraumeni JF (eds) Cancer epidemiology and prevention. Oxford University Press, New York, pp 946–958

Moolgavkar SH, Meza R, Turim J (2009) Pleural and peritoneal mesotheliomas in SEER: age effects and temporal trends, 1973–2005. Cancer Causes Control 20:935–944

Mueller N, Grufferman S (2006) Hodgkin lymphoma. In: Schottenfeld D, Fraumeni JF (eds) Cancer epidemiology and prevention. Oxford University Press, New York, pp 872–897

Naldi L, Gallus S, Tavani A, Imberti GL, La Vecchia C (2004) Risk of melanoma and vitamin A, coffee and alcohol: a case-control study from Italy. Eur J Cancer Prev 13:503–508

Negri E, Ron E, Franceschi S, La Vecchia C, Preston-Martin S, Kolonel L et al (2002) Risk factors for medullary thyroid carcinoma: a pooled analysis. Cancer Causes Control 13:365–372

Negri E, Pelucchi C, Franceschi S, Montella M, Conti E, Dal Maso L et al (2003) Family history of cancer and risk of ovarian cancer. Eur J Cancer 39:505–510

Negri E, Pelucchi C, Talamini R, Montella M, Gallus S, Bosetti C et al (2005) Family history of cancer and the risk of prostate cancer and benign prostatic hyperplasia. Int J Cancer 114:648–652

Olshan F (2006) Cancer of the larynx. In: Schottenfeld D, Fraumeni JF (eds) Cancer epidemiology and prevention. Oxford University Press, New York, pp 627–637

Palmer J, Feltmate C (2006) Choriocarcinoma. In: Schottenfeld D, Fraumeni JF (eds) Cancer epidemiology and prevention, vol 3. Oxford University Press, New York, pp 1075–1086

Parkin DM (2006) The global health burden of infection-associated cancers in the year 2002. Int J Cancer 118:3030–3044

Parkin DM, Whelan SL, Ferlay J, Teppo L, Thomas DB (eds) (2002) Cancer incidence in five continents, vol VIII. IARC Scientific Publications No. 155, IARC, Lyon

Pelucchi C, Bosetti C, Negri E, Malvezzi M, La Vecchia C (2006) Mechanisms of disease: the epidemiology of bladder cancer. Nat Clin Pract Urol 3:327–340

Pelucchi C, Galeone C, Talamini R, Bosetti C, Montella M, Negri E et al (2007) Lifetime ovulatory cycles and ovarian cancer risk in 2 Italian case-control studies. Am J Obstet Gynecol 196(83):e81–e87

Pelucchi C, Bosetti C, Rossi M, Negri E, La Vecchia C (2009) Selected aspects of Mediterranean diet and cancer risk. Nutr Cancer 61:756–766

Pelucchi C, Tramacere I, Boffetta P, Negri E, La Vecchia C (2011) Alcohol consumption and cancer risk. Nutr Cancer 63:983–990

Peng S, Lu B, Ruan W, Zhu Y, Sheng H, Lai M (2011) Genetic polymorphisms and breast cancer risk: evidence from meta-analyses, pooled analyses, and genome-wide association studies. Breast Cancer Res Treat 127:309–324

Peters U, Jiao S, Schumacher FR, Hutter CM, Aragaki AK, Baron JA et al (2013) Identification of genetic susceptibility loci for colorectal tumors in a genome-wide meta-analysis. Gastroenterology 144(799–807):e724

Peto R (1977) Epidemiology, multistage models and short-term mutagenicity tests. In: Hiatt HH, Watson JD, Winsten JA (eds) Origins of human cancer. Cold Spring Harbor, Cold Spring Harbor Laboratory, pp 1403–1428

Peto J (2012) That the effects of smoking should be measured in pack-years: misconceptions 4. Br J Cancer 107:406–407

Peto J, Seidman H, Selikoff IJ (1982) Mesothelioma mortality in asbestos workers: implications for models of carcinogenesis and risk assessment. Br J Cancer 45:124–135

Peto R, Gray R, Brantom P, Grasso P (1991) Effects on 4080 rats of chronic ingestion of N-nitrosodiethylamine or N-nitrosodimethylamine: a detailed dose-response study. Cancer Res 51:6415–6451

Peto J, Decarli A, La Vecchia C, Levi F, Negri E (1999) The European mesothelioma epidemic. Br J Cancer 79:666–672

Peto R, Darby S, Deo H, Silcocks P, Whitley E, Doll R (2000) Smoking, smoking cessation, and lung cancer in the UK since 1950: combination of national statistics with two case-control studies. BMJ 321:323–329

Pettersson A, Richiardi L, Nordenskjold A, Kaijser M, Akre O (2007) Age at surgery for undescended testis and risk of testicular cancer. N Engl J Med 356:1835–1841

Pira E, Pelucchi C, Piolatto PG, Negri E, Discalzi G, La Vecchia C (2007) First and subsequent asbestos exposures in relation to mesothelioma and lung cancer mortality. Br J Cancer 97: 1300–1304

Pirie K, Peto R, Reeves GK, Green J, Beral V (2013) The 21st century hazards of smoking and benefits of stopping: a prospective study of one million women in the UK. Lancet 381: 133–141

Platz E, Giovannucci E (2006) Prostate cancer. In: Schottenfeld D, Fraumeni JF (eds) Cancer epidemiology and prevention. Oxford University Press, New York, pp 1128–1150

Plummer M, Vivas J, Lopez G, Bravo JC, Peraza S, Carillo E et al (2007) Chemoprevention of precancerous gastric lesions with antioxidant vitamin supplementation: a randomized trial in a high-risk population. J Natl Cancer Inst 99:137–146

Plummer M, Peto J, Franceschi S (2012) Time since first sexual intercourse and the risk of cervical cancer. Int J Cancer 130:2638–2644

Preston-Martin S, Munir R, Chakrabarti I (2006) Nervous system. In: Schottenfeld D, Fraumeni JF (eds) Cancer epidemiology and prevention. Oxford University Press, New York, pp 1173–1195

Randi G, Franceschi S, La Vecchia C (2006) Gallbladder cancer worldwide: geographical distribution and risk factors. Int J Cancer 118:1591–1602

Rizzato C, Campa D, Pezzilli R, Soucek P, Greenhalf W, Capurso G et al (2013) ABO blood groups and pancreatic cancer risk and survival: results from the PANcreatic Disease ReseArch (PANDoRA) consortium. Oncol Rep 29:1637–1644

Ron E, Schneider A (2006) Thyroid cancer. In: Schottenfeld D, Fraumeni JF (eds) Cancer epidemiology and prevention. Oxford University Press, New York, pp 975–994

Ross J, Spector L (2006) Cancers in children. In: Schottenfeld D, Fraumeni JF (eds) Cancer epidemiology and prevention. Oxford University Press, New York, pp 1251–1268

Rothwell PM, Fowkes FG, Belch JF, Ogawa H, Warlow CP, Meade TW (2011) Effect of daily aspirin on long-term risk of death due to cancer: analysis of individual patient data from randomised trials. Lancet 377:31–41

Sankaranarayanan R, Swaminathan R, Jayant K, Brenner H (2011) An overview of cancer survival in Africa, Asia, the Caribbean and Central America: the case for investment in cancer health services. IARC Sci Publ (162):257–291

Sankaranarayanan R, Ramadas K, Thara S, Muwonge R, Thomas G, Anju G et al (2013) Long term effect of visual screening on oral cancer incidence and mortality in a randomized trial in Kerala, India. Oral Oncol 49:314–321

Sant M, Allemani C, Santaquilani M, Knijn A, Marchesi F, Capocaccia R (2009) EUROCARE-4. Survival of cancer patients diagnosed in 1995–1999. Results and commentary. Eur J Cancer 45:931–991

Sanyal AJ, Yoon SK, Lencioni R (2010) The etiology of hepatocellular carcinoma and consequences for treatment. Oncologist 15(suppl 4):14–22

Sarma A, McLaughlin J, Schottenfeld D (2006) Testicular cancer. In: Schottenfeld D, Fraumeni JF (eds) Cancer epidemiology and prevention. Oxford University Press, New York, pp 1151–1165

Schiffman M, Hildesheim A (2006) Cervical cancer. In: Schottenfeld D, Fraumeni JF (eds) Cancer epidemiology and prevention. Oxford University Press, New York, pp 1044–1067

Schottenfeld D, Beebe-Dimmer JL, Buffler PA, Omenn GS (2013) Current perspective on the global and United States cancer burden attributable to lifestyle and environmental risk factors. Annu Rev Public Health 34:97–117

Shah KV (2007) SV40 and human cancer: a review of recent data. Int J Cancer 120:215–223

Sigurdsson JA, Getz L, Sjonell G, Vainiomaki P, Brodersen J (2013) Marginal public health gain of screening for colorectal cancer: modelling study, based on WHO and national databases in the Nordic countries. J Eval Clin Pract 19:400–407

Silverman D, Devesa S, Moore L, Rothman N (2006) Bladder cancer. In: Schottenfeld D, Fraumeni JF (eds) Cancer epidemiology and prevention. Oxford University Press, New York, pp 1101–1127

Smith JS, Lindsay L, Hoots B, Keys J, Franceschi S, Winer R et al (2007) Human papillomavirus type distribution in invasive cervical cancer and high-grade cervical lesions: a meta-analysis update. Int J Cancer 121:621–632

Smith RA, Brooks D, Cokkinides V, Saslow D, Brawley OW (2013) Cancer screening in the United States, 2013: a review of current American Cancer Society guidelines, current issues in cancer screening, and new guidance on cervical cancer screening and lung cancer screening. CA Cancer J Clin 63:88–105

Soerjomataram I, Lortet-Tieulent J, Parkin DM, Ferlay J, Mathers C, Forman D et al (2012) Global burden of cancer in 2008: a systematic analysis of disability-adjusted life-years in 12 world regions. Lancet 380:1840–1850

Song Y, Zhao L, Palipudi KM, Asma S, Morton J, Talley B et al (2013) Tracking MPOWER in 14 countries: results from the Global Adult Tobacco Survey, 2008–2010. Glob Health Promot PMID 24042973

Stadler ZK, Thom P, Robson ME, Weitzel JN, Kauff ND, Hurley KE et al (2010) Genome-wide association studies of cancer. J Clin Oncol 28:4255–4267

Stefanick ML, Anderson GL, Margolis KL, Hendrix SL, Rodabough RJ, Paskett ED et al (2006) Effects of conjugated equine estrogens on breast cancer and mammography screening in postmenopausal women with hysterectomy. JAMA 295:1647–1657

Steinmaus CM, Ferreccio C, Romo JA, Yuan Y, Cortes S, Marshall G et al (2013) Drinking water arsenic in northern Chile: high cancer risks 40 years after exposure cessation. Cancer Epidemiol Biomarkers Prev 22:623–630

Tang M, Lautenberger JA, Gao X, Sezgin E, Hendrickson SL, Troyer JL et al (2012) The principal genetic determinants for nasopharyngeal carcinoma in China involve the HLA class I antigen recognition groove. PLoS Genet 8:e1003103

Tramacere I, Scotti L, Jenab M, Bagnardi V, Bellocco R, Rota M et al (2010) Alcohol drinking and pancreatic cancer risk: a meta-analysis of the dose-risk relation. Int J Cancer 126:1474–1486

Tramacere I, La Vecchia C, Negri E (2011) Tobacco smoking and esophageal and gastric cardia adenocarcinoma: a meta-analysis. Epidemiology 22:344–349

Tramacere I, Pelucchi C, Bagnardi V, Rota M, Scotti L, Islami F et al (2012) A meta-analysis on alcohol drinking and esophageal and gastric cardia adenocarcinoma risk. Ann Oncol 23: 287–297

Trichopoulos D (1990) Hypothesis: does breast cancer originate in utero? Lancet 335:939–940

Truong T, Hung RJ, Amos CI, Wu X, Bickeboller H, Rosenberger A et al (2010) Replication of lung cancer susceptibility loci at chromosomes 15q25, 5p15, and 6p21: a pooled analysis from the International Lung Cancer Consortium. J Natl Cancer Inst 102:959–971

Turati F, Talamini R, Pelucchi C, Polesel J, Franceschi S, Crispo A et al (2013a) Metabolic syndrome and hepatocellular carcinoma risk. Br J Cancer 108:222–228

Turati F, Tramacere I, La Vecchia C, Negri E (2013b) A meta-analysis of body mass index and esophageal and gastric cardia adenocarcinoma. Ann Oncol 24:609–617

Urayama KY, Chokkalingam AP, Metayer C, Ma X, Selvin S, Barcellos LF et al (2012) HLA-DP genetic variation, proxies for early life immune modulation and childhood acute lymphoblastic leukemia risk. Blood 120:3039–3047

Vineis P, Manuguerra M, Kavvoura FK, Guarrera S, Allione A, Rosa F et al (2009) A field synopsis on low-penetrance variants in DNA repair genes and cancer susceptibility. J Natl Cancer Inst 101:24–36

WCRF (2007) World Cancer Research Fund/American Institute for Cancer Research. Food, nutrition, physical activity, and the prevention of cancer: a global perspective. AICR, Washington, DC

Welch HG, Albertsen PC (2009) Prostate cancer diagnosis and treatment after the introduction of prostate-specific antigen screening: 1986–2005. J Natl Cancer Inst 101:1325–1329

WHO (1990) International classification of diseases for oncology (ICD-O), 2nd edn. World Health Organization, Geneva

Widerof fL, Schottenfeld D (2006) Penile cancer. In: Schottenfeld D, Fraumeni JF (eds) Cancer epidemiology and prevention. Oxford University Press, New York, pp 1166–1172

Wu S, Feng B, Li K, Zhu X, Liang S, Liu X et al (2012) Fish consumption and colorectal cancer risk in humans: a systematic review and meta-analysis. Am J Med 125:551–559.e5

Yeager M, Orr N, Hayes RB, Jacobs KB, Kraft P, Wacholder S et al (2007) Genome-wide association study of prostate cancer identifies a second risk locus at 8q24. Nat Genet 39:645–649

Yu M, Yuan J (2006) Nasopharyngeal cancer. In: Schottenfeld D, Fraumeni JF (eds) Cancer epidemiology and prevention. Oxford University Press, New York, pp 620–626

Zendehdel K, Nyren O, Luo J, Dickman PW, Boffetta P, Englund A et al (2008) Risk of gastroesophageal cancer among smokers and users of Scandinavian moist snuff. Int J Cancer 122:1095–1099

Zhang Z-F, Boffetta P, Neugut AI, La Vecchia C (2014) Cancer epidemiology and public health. In: Oxford textbook of public health. Oxford University Press, Oxford

Printed by Publishers' Graphics LLC